Ketogenic Diet And Cookbook

A Complete Guide To Ketogenic Healthy Diet

[Michelle J. Griffin]

Text Copyright ©

Legal & Disclaimer

all risks of using the information presented inside this book. You agree that by continuing to read this book, where appropriate and necessary, you shall consult a professional (including but not limited to your doctor, attorney, or financial advisor, or such other advisor as needed) before using any of the suggested remedies, techniques, or information in this book.

Table Of Contents

Introduction

What is the Ketogenic Diet?

The ketogenic diet is a special diet intended to support children with epilepsy who do not adapt appropriately to common anti-epileptic drugs. The standard ketogenic diet consists of the following:

- ✓ Adequate levels of protein
- ✓ A high proportion of fats
- ✓ A low proportion of carbohydrates

This diet is called ketogenic because it mimics fasting symptoms, which allows the body to create ketones. During malnutrition, the body is forced to burn fat rather than starch. In a ketogenic diet, fat is the primary source of calories, and when it is combined with reduced consumption of carbohydrates, the body makes ketones. When a human eats a daily diet, the food is converted to glucose, which is then transferred throughout the body and used as an energy supply for different cells. The brain typically depends on glucose as an energy supply. When minimal carbs are available, the liver processes fats to provide energy to the brain in fatty acids and ketones. Increased ketone bodies' blood levels are referred to as ketosis, and some studies have found that ketogenic diets are associated with seizure reduction in children with epilepsy that is difficult to handle. The ketogenic diet provides ample quantities of protein for body development and repair. Therefore, total calories in the diet are necessary to sustain a good weight at a given age and height. The ketogenic (keto) diet is a low-carb and high-fat diet that offers many comparisons with the low-carb diets and Atkins. It includes drastically decreasing carbohydrate intake and then replacing it with fat. This modification in carbs sets our body in a metabolic state, and it is called ketosis. When it occurs, our body converts strangely efficient at consuming fat for energy. It also converts fat into ketones in our liver, which can provide power to the brain. These diets can create considerable losses in insulin levels and blood sugar. A keto (ketogenic) diet is a low-carb, balanced protein, a higher-fat diet that can support you burn fat more efficiently. It has multiple benefits for health, weight loss, and performance, as proved in over 50 studies.

For this reason, it has been suggested by so many doctors. It can be beneficial for dropping excess body fat without hunger and developing type 2 diabetes. It is a low-carb and high-fat diet that contributes to many health benefits. It may even have advantages against epilepsy, diabetes, cancer, and Alzheimer's disease.

Why is the keto diet right for you?

A keto diet is a meal plan that emphasizes ingredients that have a lot of healthier fats, sufficient levels of protein, and relatively little carbs. The target is to get more calories from fat than from carbohydrates. The diet works by depleting the body's sugar supplies. As a consequence, it's going to begin to break down fat for energy. This results in the creation of molecules called ketones, which the body uses for food. When the body loses fat, it can also contribute to weight loss. There are many types of the keto diet, including the Regular Ketogenic Diet and the Cyclic Ketogenic Diet. The advantages of the keto diet are as follows:

1. **Supports Weight Loss:** Ketogenic diets can help facilitate weight loss in various areas, including improving metabolism and decreasing appetite. Ketogenic diets consist of foods that fill a person and can suppress hunger-stimulating hormones. For these reasons, a keto diet can reduce the need and promote weight loss. In a 2013 meta-analysis of 13 separate randomized clinical trials, researchers observed that individuals with ketogenic diets lost 2 pounds (lbs) more than those with low-fat diets over one year. Similarly, another

review of 11 studies demonstrated that people following a ketogenic diet lost 5 kg more than those following low-fat diets after six months.

2. **Improves Acne:** Acne has various common causes that can be linked with food and blood sugar in certain people. Eating a diet high in processed and refined carbohydrates can alter the composition of the intestinal bacteria and cause blood sugar to rise and fall dramatically, all of which can adversely affect the skin's health.

3. **May Reduce Risk Of Certain Cancers:** Researchers also studied the effects of ketogenic diets on avoiding or even treating some cancers. One research showed a ketogenic diet could be a healthy and appropriate alternative treatment for chemotherapy and radiation therapy in patients with some cancers. This is because it can induce more oxidative stress in cancer cells than normal cells, allowing them to die. More recent research in 2018 indicates that because the ketogenic diet lowers blood sugar, the likelihood of diabetes complications may also be reduced. Insulin is a chemical that regulates blood sugar and can be related to some cancers. While some research suggests that ketogenic diets may benefit the treatment of cancer, there are limited studies in this area. Researchers need further research to truly understand the ketogenic diet's possible effects on cancer prevention and care.

4. **May Improve Heart Health:** When a person follows a ketogenic diet, it is crucial that they chose nutritious foods. There is evidence that consuming healthy fats, such as avocados, instead of less healthy fats, such as pork rinds, will help boost heart health by lowering cholesterol. A 2017 analysis of animal and human keto diet trials found that specific individuals observed a substantial reduction in total cholesterol, low-density lipoprotein (LDL), or low cholesterol and triglyceride levels and a rise in high-density lipoprotein (HDL) or "good" cholesterol. High levels of cholesterol can increase the risk of cardiovascular disease. Decreasing the

impact of the keto diet on cholesterol may also reduce the risk of heart problems for an individual.

Ketogenic Diets Can Help to Lose Weight

A ketogenic diet is a useful way to lower risk factors for disease and lose weight. Research explains that the ketogenic diet is significantly superior to the regularly suggested low-fat diet. The menu is so fulfilling that you can properly lose weight without calculating calories or following your food intake. Some studies discovered that people on a ketogenic diet lost (2.2) times more weight than those on a calorie-restricted (low-fat) diet. HDL cholesterol and Triglyceride levels also developed. Another study discovered that people touching the ketogenic diet dropped three times more extra weight than those at the diet suggested by Diabetes UK. Also, there are many causes why this diet is excellent to a low-fat menu, including the enhanced protein consumption, which gives numerous advantages. The improved ketones, lower blood sugar levels, and increased insulin responsiveness may also present a key role.

Ketogenic Diets for Diabetes and Prediabetes

Diabetes has defined by changes in metabolism, impaired insulin function, and high blood sugar. The ketogenic diet can help you lose excess fat, which is precisely linked to type 2 diabetes, metabolic syndrome, and prediabetes. One study discovered that the ketogenic diet developed insulin responsiveness by a whopping 75%. A different study in people with type 2 diabetes noticed that 7 of the 21 members could prevent utilizing all diabetes medications. In another research, the ketogenic group wasted (24.4 pounds /11.1 kg), related to (15.2 pounds /6.9 kg) in the higher-carb group. It is a significant advantage when considering the link between weight and type two diabetes.

95.2% of the ketogenic-group were adequately able to stop diabetes medication, matched to 63% in the higher-carb group.

Other Health Benefits of Keto

The ketogenic diet is introduced as a tool for managing neurological diseases like epilepsy. Researchers have now proved that the diet can have advantages for a wide variety of various health conditions:

1) **Cancer:** This diet is currently being practiced to treat different types of slow tumor growth and cancer.
2) **Heart Disease:** It can improve risk factors like body fat, blood pressure, blood sugar, and HDL cholesterol levels.
3) **Alzheimer's Disease:** It may reduce the signs of Alzheimer's disease and properly slow its progression.
4) **Parkinson's Disease:** Some studies discovered that the diet helped to improve the symptoms of Parkinson's disease.
5) **Epilepsy:** Some research has explained that this diet can cause massive decreases in convulsions in epileptic children.
6) **Polycystic Ovary Syndrome:** This diet can reduce our insulin levels, which may play a vital role in polycystic ovary syndrome.
7) **Acne:** Eating less sugar and lower insulin levels may help to promote acne.
8) **Brain Injuries:** A animal study discovered that the diet could decrease concussions and aid recovery after the brain injury.

Different Types of Ketogenic Diets

There are different versions of the ketogenic diet, including:

A Cyclical Ketogenic Diet (CKD): Ketogenic diet combines periods of the higher-carb refeeds, like five ketogenic days followed by two high-carb days.

A Standard Ketogenic Diet (SKD): Ketogenic diet is a very moderate-protein, high-fat, and low-carb. It typically combines 20% protein, 75% fat, and only 5% carbs.

High-protein Ketogenic Diet: It is related to a regular ketogenic diet but includes more protein. Its ratio is often 35% protein, 60% fat, and 5% carbs.

A Targeted Ketogenic Diet (TKD): Ketogenic diet permits you to combine carbs approximately workouts.

How the Keto Diet Works

The ketogenic diet is a high fat, moderate protein, low carbohydrate eating pattern, which varies from the general, balanced eating guidelines. Many nutrient-rich foods are carbohydrate sources, like berries, plants, whole grains, milk, and yogurt. Carbs from all types are heavily limited in the keto diet. To maintain carbohydrates below 50 grams a day, keto dieters often eat no bread, grain, or cereals. And even fruit and vegetables are limited since they often contain carbohydrates. For most people, the keto diet needs a significant change in how they usually consume.

Why does the Keto diet restrict carbs?

Carbs are our body's primary source of nutrition. The body breaks down fat into ketones without enough carbohydrates for nutrition. The ketones would then become the primary source of food for the body. Ketones supply energy to the heart, kidneys, and other muscles. The body also uses ketones as an alternate form of nutrition for the brain. So the name for this eating pattern. In reality, a ketogenic diet is a partial fast for our bodies. In a completely fast or starving state, the body has no supply of nutrition. It breaks down the lean muscle mass for heat. The ketone diet offers an alternative source of sugar. Unlike an easy, keto diet tends to preserve lean muscle mass.

Some Keto Foods

Here is a collection of all low-carb, keto-friendly things that you can consume while you practice keto.

- Fish and seafood
- Cheese
- Low-carb veggies
- Avocados
- Dark chocolate and cocoa powder
- Eggs
- poultry
- Nuts, seeds, and healthful oils
- Berries
- Plain Greek yogurt and cottage cheese
- Unsweetened coffee and tea

List of Foods You Can't Eat on the Keto Diet

- ➢ Starchy vegetables and high-sugar fruits
- ➢ Grains
- ➢ Sweetened yogurt
- ➢ Baked goods, including gluten-free baked goods
- ➢ Honey, syrup, or sugar in any form
- ➢ Juices
- ➢ Chips and crackers

RECIPES

RECIPES

Garlic Tuscan Chicken

Preparation Time: *20 Minutes Yield: 1 Serving*

Ingredients

- Two tablespoons olive oil
- 1/2 pounds skinless, boneless chicken breasts
- 1 cup heavy cream
- 1 or 2 cups of chicken broth
- 1 or 2 cups grated Parmesan cheese
- One teaspoon garlic powder
- One teaspoon Italian seasoning
- 1 cup spinach, chopped
- 1/2 cup sun-dried tomatoes

Directions

- First, heat the olive oil properly in a medium skillet over medium-high temperature. Cook chicken until browned and no longer pink in the center, 3 to 5 minutes per side. Separate chicken and set it aside on a plate.
- Combine heavy cream, chicken broth, Parmesan cheese, garlic powder, and Italian seasoning to the skillet. Whisk the sauce over medium-high heat until starting to thicken, about 10 minutes. Add spinach and sun-dried tomatoes; simmer until the spinach begins to wilt, about 1 minute. Return the chicken to the skillet and cook it until heated for 2 to 3 minutes.

Nutrition's Fact: Calories 215, Carbohydrates 25g, Protein 36g, Fat 2g

Keto Chicken Parmesan

Preparation Time: *20 Minutes Yield: 1 Serving*

Ingredients

- 1 (8 ounces) skinless, boneless chicken breast
- One egg
- One tablespoon heavy whipping cream
- 1 1/2 ounces pork rinds, crushed
- 1 ounce grated Parmesan cheese
- 1/2 teaspoon salt
- 1/2 teaspoon garlic powder
- 1/2 teaspoon red pepper flakes (optional)
- 1/2 teaspoon ground black pepper
- 1/2 teaspoon Italian seasoning
- 1/2 cup jarred tomato sauce
- 1/4 cup shredded mozzarella cheese
- One tablespoon ghee

Directions

- First, Set an oven rack properly about 5 inches from the heat source and preheat the oven's broiler.
- Slice chicken breast through the center horizontally from one side to within 1 or 2 inches of the other hand. Remove the two sides and spread them out like an open book — pound chicken flat until about one or 2-inch thick.
- Then beat the cream and egg together in a bowl.
- Mix the Parmesan cheese, salt, crushed pork rinds, garlic powder, red pepper flakes, ground black pepper, and Italian seasoning in a bowl; a transfer is breading to a plate.

- Dip chicken into egg mixture; coat thoroughly. Press the chicken into breading; thickly coat both sides.
- Heat a skillet over medium-high temperature; add ghee. Place chicken in the pan; cook it until no longer pink in the center, and the juices run free, about 5 minutes per side. An instant-read thermometer adequately inserted into the middle should read at least 165 degrees F. Be careful to keep breading in place.
- Transfer the chicken to a baking sheet. Cover it with tomato sauce; top with mozzarella cheese.
- Broil it until cheese is bubbling and barely browned for about 2 minutes.

Nutrition's Fact: Calories 260, Carbohydrates 18g, Protein 30g, Fat 2g

Sausage, Zucchini, and Cauli Keto Risotto

Preparation Time: *20 Minutes Yield: 1 Serving*

Ingredients

- 1/4 cup ghee
- 1/2 onion, finely chopped
- One clove garlic, minced
- Two links chicken sausage
- One head cauliflower, grated
- 1/2 zucchini, sliced
- 1/2 cup heavy whipping cream
- 1 cup grated Parmesan cheese
- 1/2 teaspoon salt
- 1/4 teaspoon ground black pepper
- 1/4 teaspoon ground nutmeg

Directions

- Melt the ghee properly in a skillet over medium temperature. Combine onion and garlic; cook until tender, about 5 minutes. Stir it in sausage and grated cauliflower; cook it for 5 minutes more. Combine zucchini and cook until tender, about 5 minutes.
- Stir heavy cream, Parmesan cheese, salt, pepper, and nutmeg into the skillet; cook over medium heat until creamy, 6 to 7 minutes.

Nutrition's Fact: Calories 261, Carbohydrates 17g, Protein 31g, Fat 5g

Keto Beef Egg Roll Slaw

Preparation Time: *20 Minutes Yield: 1 Serving*

Ingredients

- Two tablespoons sesame oil
- 1/2 cup diced onion
- Five green onions, chopped
- Three cloves garlic, minced
- 1 1/2 pounds ground beef
- One tablespoon chili-garlic sauce
- 1/2 teaspoon ground ginger
- sea salt to taste
- ground black pepper to taste
- 1 (14 ounces) package coleslaw mix
- Three tablespoons soy sauce
- One tablespoon apple cider vinegar

Directions

- First, heat the oil in a medium skillet over medium-high temperature. Add white parts of the green onions, diced onion, and garlic. Saute the onions continuously are translucent, and garlic is fragrant for about 10 minutes. Add sriracha, ginger, salt, ground beef, and black pepper. Saute until the meat is browned and crumbly, about 10 minutes.
- Stir soy sauce, coleslaw mix, and cider vinegar into the beef mix. Saute until coleslaw is tender, about 5 minutes more. Top with the rest of the green onions.

Nutrition's Fact: Calories 263, Carbohydrates 19g, Protein 33g, Fat 1g

Keto Smoky Chicken With Vegetable

Preparation Time: *20 Minutes Yield: 1 Serving*

Ingredients

- One head broccoli
- 1 or 2 head cauliflower florets
- 1 or 2 medium head red cabbage
- 1 or 2 cup olive oil
- One teaspoon of sea salt
- One teaspoon smoked paprika
- One tablespoon chili powder
- One teaspoon cumin
- One teaspoon garlic powder
- Four boneless, skinless chicken thighs
- Eight slices bacon

Directions

- Preheat the oven carefully to 400 degrees F (200 degrees C). Line a baking sheet with aluminum foil.
- Mix the cauliflower, broccoli, and cabbage in a bowl. Whisk olive oil, salt, and paprika mutually in a measuring cup and pour over vegetables. Smoothly stir until all of the herbs have coated. Set aside.
- Combine cumin, chili powder, and garlic powder on a flat plate. Roll each chicken thigh in the spice mix so that both sides have coated. Wrap two bacon pieces around each leg and place the chicken in the middle of the baking sheet.
- Stir vegetables one last time and scatter them around the chicken in an even layer.

- Bake it in the preheated oven until bacon is crispy and chicken is no longer pink in the middle properly, and the juices run clear for 45 minutes. An instant-read thermometer entered into the center should read at least 165 degrees F.

Nutrition's Fact: Calories 262, Carbohydrates 21g, Protein 34g, Fat 4g

Creamy Keto Cauliflower Risotto

Preparation Time: *20 Minutes Yield: 1 Serving*

Ingredients

- 1/4 cup ghee
- 1/2 onion, finely chopped
- One clove garlic, minced
- One head cauliflower, grated
- 1 cup sliced fresh mushrooms
- 1/2 cup heavy whipping cream
- 1 cup grated Parmesan cheese
- 1/2 teaspoon salt
- 1/4 teaspoon ground black pepper
- 1/4 teaspoon ground nutmeg

Directions

- Melt the ghee in a skillet over average temperature. Add garlic and onion; cook it until tender, about 5 minutes. Stir in grated cauliflower; cook for 5 minutes more. Combine mushrooms and cook it until tender, about 5 minutes.
- Stir heavy cream, Parmesan cheese, salt, pepper, and nutmeg into the skillet; cook over medium heat until creamy, 6 to 8 minutes.

Nutrition's Fact: Calories 264, Carbohydrates 22g, Protein 31g, Fat 6g

Creamy Keto Taco Soup with Ground Beef

Preparation Time: *20 Minutes Yield: 1 Serving*

Ingredients

- 1 pound ground beef
- 1/2 cup chopped onion
- Two cloves garlic, minced
- One tablespoon ground cumin
- One teaspoon chili powder
- 1 (8 ounces) package cream cheese, softened
- 14.5 ounces beef broth
- 10 ounce diced tomatoes and green chiles
- 1/2 cup heavy cream
- Two teaspoons salt, or to taste

Directions

- Combine the ground beef properly with garlic and onion in a large soup pot over medium-high heat. Cook it and then stir it until the meat has browned and crumbly, 6 to 8 minutes. Drain and discard grease. Combine cumin and chili powder; cook 5 minutes also.
- Drop the cream cheese inside the pot by bits and mash it properly into the beef with a spoon until no white spots remain 10 minutes. Stir it in heavy cream, broth, diced tomatoes, and salt. Cook it until heated through, about 10 minutes more.

Nutrition's Fact: Calories 268, Carbohydrates 24g, Protein 33g, Fat 3g

Keto Smothered Chicken Thighs

Preparation Time: *20 Minutes Yield: 1 Serving*

Ingredients

- 4 (8 ounces) skin-on, bone-in chicken thighs
- One teaspoon paprika
- salt and pepper to taste
- Four slices bacon, cut into 1/2 inch pieces
- 1/3 cup low-sodium chicken broth
- 4 ounces sliced mushrooms
- 1/4 cup heavy whipping cream
- Two green onions, white and green parts, separated and sliced

Directions

- Preheat the oven properly to 400 degrees F.
- Season the chicken thighs properly on each side with paprika, salt, and pepper.
- Cook bacon in a cast-iron skillet or oven-safe pan over medium-high temperature until browned, 5 to 6 minutes. Separate it from the skillet and drain it on a paper towel-lined plate. Drain and discard excess grease from skillet.
- Return skillet to medium temperature and cook chicken thighs, skin-side down, for 5 to 6 minutes: Flip the chicken over and place skillet in the preheated oven.
- Bake it until chicken thighs are no longer pink at the bone and juices run clear, about 35 minutes. Remove the chicken to a plate and cover it adequately with foil to keep it warm. Remove all but two tablespoons of drippings from the skillet.
- Return to the skillet to the stove over medium-high temperature. Pour in chicken broth while fluttering up brown

bits from the bottom of the skillet. Add mushrooms and cook it until soft, about 5 to 6 minutes. Pour it in heavy whipping cream and whisk together until lightly simmering, then reduce heat to medium-low. Season with salt and pepper, if necessary.

- Return chicken and any juices into skillet; top with bacon and green onions. Serve immediately, spooning sauce over the chicken.

Nutrition's Fact: Calories 265, Carbohydrates 22g, Protein 29g, Fat 5g

Ultimate Low-Carb Zucchini Lasagna

Preparation Time: *20 Minutes Yield: 1 Serving*

Ingredients

- cooking spray
- 1 1/2 large zucchinis, thinly sliced lengthwise
- One tablespoon olive oil
- 1 pound ground beef
- 1 1/2 cups low-carb marinara sauce
- Two teaspoons salt, divided
- One teaspoon dried oregano
- 1/2 teaspoon ground black pepper
- 1 (8 ounces) container ricotta cheese
- One egg
- 1/2 teaspoon ground nutmeg
- 2 cups shredded mozzarella cheese, divided
- 1/4 cup grated Parmesan cheese

Directions

- First, preheat the oven carefully to 375 degrees F or 190 degrees C. Grease an 8-inch baking dish with cooking spray.
- Pat dry the zucchini slices with a paper towel to get rid of excess moisture.
- Heat the olive oil carefully in a saucepan over medium-high heat. Add ground beef; cook until browned, 5 to 8 minutes. Add marinara sauce, one teaspoon salt, oregano, and pepper; simmer for 10 minutes.
- Combine the remaining one teaspoon salt, ricotta cheese, egg, and nutmeg in a bowl; mix well.

- Make one layer of zucchini slices in the prepared baking dish. Cover with 1/2 of the sauce. Add another layer of zucchini slices. Spread the ricotta mix on top sprinkle with 1 cup mozzarella cheese. Add another layer of zucchini slices; cover with the remaining sauce and top with 1 cup mozzarella cheese and Parmesan cheese. Cover baking dish with aluminum foil.
- Finally, bake it properly in the preheated oven for 35 minutes. Remove aluminum foil and cook until the top is golden, about 15 minutes more.

Nutrition's Fact: Calories 264, Carbohydrates 20g, Protein 35g, Fat 4g

Keto Chicken and Kale Stew

Preparation Time: *20 Minutes Yield: 1 Serving*

Ingredients

- One tablespoon butter
- 1/2 onion, chopped
- Two boneless chicken breasts, diced
- 1 (14.5 ounces) can diced tomatoes
- 3 cups chopped kale
- 1 cup chicken broth
- 1/2 teaspoon salt
- 1/2 teaspoon garlic powder
- 1/2 teaspoon oregano
- 1/4 teaspoon ground black pepper

Directions

- Turn on a pressure cooker and select the Saute function. Melt butter and cook onion until soft and tender, about 5 minutes. Add chicken; cook it until golden and crispy, about 5 minutes.
- Place the salt, garlic powder, oregano, diced tomatoes, kale, chicken broth, and black pepper in the pot.
- Close and lock the lid properly. Select the high pressure according to the manufacturer's directions; set the timer for 15 minutes. Allow 10 minutes for pressure to build.
- Release the pressure properly using the natural-release system according to the manufacturer's instructions, about 15 minutes.
- Complete the releasing trouble carefully using the quick-release system according to the manufacturer's instructions, about 6 minutes. Unlock and remove the lid.

Nutrition's Fact: Calories 261, Carbohydrates 19g, Protein 31g, Fat 3g

Keto Brownies

Preparation Time: *20 Minutes Yield: 1 Serving*

Ingredients

- 3 or 4 cups of cocoa powder
- 1 or 2 teaspoon baking soda
- 2 or 3 cup coconut oil, divided
- 1 or 2 cups boiling water
- 1 cup stevia sugar substitute
- Two eggs
- 1 1/3 cups almond flour
- One teaspoon vanilla extract
- 1/4 teaspoon salt

Directions

- First, preheat the oven carefully to 350 degrees F. Lightly grease an 8-inch square pan spontaneously with coconut oil.
- Whisk the cocoa powder and baking soda together in a bowl. Add 1 or 3 cup coconut oil and boiling water; mix until well blended. Add remaining 1 or 3 cup stevia, coconut oil, and eggs; blend properly. Fold vanilla extract, almond flour, and salt into the batter.
- Pour the batter into the greased pan.
- Bake it properly in the preheated oven until the top is dry and edges have started to properly pull away from the pan's surfaces, 35 to 45 minutes. Let cool before cutting into 12 squares.

Nutrition's Fact: Calories 215, Carbohydrates 25g, Protein 36g, Fat 2g

Basic Keto Cheese Crisps

Preparation Time: *20 Minutes Yield: 1 Serving*

Ingredients

- 1 cup shredded Cheddar cheese

Directions

- Preheat the oven carefully to 400 degrees F. Line the two baking sheets accurately with the parchment paper.
- Prepare the Cheddar cheese in 24 small heaps on the prepared baking sheets.
- Then bake it smoothly in the preheated oven until golden brown, about 7 minutes. Cold it for 5 to 10 minutes before removing it from baking sheets.

Nutrition's Fact: Calories 260, Carbohydrates 18g, Protein 30g, Fat 2g

Easy Keto Alfredo Sauce

Preparation Time: *20 Minutes Yield: 1 Serving*

Ingredients

- 1/2 cup unsalted butter
- Two cloves garlic, crushed
- 2 cups heavy whipping cream
- 1/2 (4 ounces) package cream cheese, softened
- 1 1/2 cups grated Parmesan cheese
- One pinch salt, or to taste
- One pinch ground nutmeg, or to taste
- One pinch ground white pepper, or to taste

Directions

- Melt butter in a medium saucepan. Cook garlic until fragrant, about 2 minutes. Add heavy cream and cream cheese. Slowly add Parmesan cheese, continually stirring until well incorporated and sauce thickens, 5 to 7 minutes. Stir in salt, nutmeg, and white pepper.

Nutrition's Fact: Calories 261, Carbohydrates 17g, Protein 31g, Fat 5g

Simple Cauliflower Keto Casserole

Preparation Time: *20 Minutes Yield: 1 Serving*

Ingredients

- 1/2 head cauliflower florets
- 1 cup shredded Cheddar cheese
- 1/2 cup heavy cream
- One pinch of salt and ground black pepper

Directions

- First, preheat the oven carefully to 450 degrees F (225 degrees C).
- Take a large pot of gently salted water to a boil and cook the cauliflower until tender but firm to the taste, about 15 minutes. Drain it.
- Combine cream, Cheddar cheese, salt, and pepper in a large bowl. Arrange the cauliflower in a casserole dish and cover with a cheese mixture.
- Bake in the preheated oven until cheese is bubbly and golden brown, about 30 minutes.

Nutrition's Fact: Calories 263, Carbohydrates 19g, Protein 33g, Fat 1g

Low-Carb Almond Cinnamon Butter Cookies

Preparation Time: *20 Minutes Yield: 1 Serving*

Ingredients

- 2 cups blanched almond flour
- 1/2 cup butter, softened
- One egg
- 1/2 cup low-calorie natural sweetener
- One teaspoon sugar-free vanilla extract
- One teaspoon ground cinnamon

Directions

- Preheat oven to 350 degrees F. Line correctly a baking sheet with parchment paper.
- Combine sweetener, vanilla extract, almond flour, butter, egg, and cinnamon in a bowl; mix it until well combined.
- Roll dough into 1-inch balls. Put it on the provided baking sheet and press down with a fork twice in a criss-cross pattern.
- Bake it in the preheated oven until the edges are golden, 15 to 16 minutes. Finally, cool it on the baking sheet for 1 minute before removing it to a wire rack to cool completely.

Nutrition's Fact: Calories 262, Carbohydrates 21g, Protein 34g, Fat 4g

Keto Low-Carb Lemon Poppy Seed Muffins

Preparation Time: *20 Minutes Yield: 1 Serving*

Ingredients

- 1 or 3 cups low-calorie natural sweetener
- 1 or 4 cups almond flour
- 1 or 4 cups of coconut flour
- One tablespoon poppy seeds
- One lemon, zested
- 1/2 teaspoon baking powder
- 1/2 teaspoon salt
- 1/4 teaspoon xanthan gum (optional)
- Three eggs
- Three tablespoons butter
- Two tablespoons sour cream
- 1/2 teaspoon vanilla extract
- Two tablespoons heavy whipping cream, or more to taste

Directions

- Preheat the oven carefully to 350 degrees F. Grease properly a muffin tin or line with paper muffin liners.
- Mix the almond flour, coconut flour, sweetener, poppy seeds, lemon zest, baking powder, salt, and xanthan gum in a bowl.
- Beat the eggs in a pot with an electric mixer on high speed until fluffy, about 5 minutes. Beat it in sour cream, butter, and vanilla extract. Add the sweetener mix. Stir it in cream gradually until the batter is thick and smooth. Pour into prepared muffin tin.
- Bake it in the preheated oven until the tops are golden, 15 to 20 minutes.

Keto Cheesecake Cupcakes

Preparation Time: *20 Minutes Yield: 1 Serving*

Ingredients

- 1/2 cup almond meal
- 1/4 cup butter, melted
- 2 (8 ounces) packages of cream cheese
- Two eggs
- 3/4 cup granular no-calorie sucralose sweetener
- One teaspoon vanilla extract

Directions

- First, preheat the oven carefully to 350 degrees F or 175 degrees C. Line the 12 muffin cups with paper liners.
- Mix almond meal and butter in a bowl; spoon it into the paper liners' bottoms and press into a flat crust.
- Beat the eggs, sweetener, cream cheese, and vanilla extract mutually in a bowl with an electric mixer set it to medium until smooth; spoon over the crust layer in the paper liners.
- Bake it properly in the preheated oven until the cream cheese mixture is almost set in the middle, 16 to 18 minutes.
- Let the cupcakes cool at room heat until cool enough to handle. Refrigerate 8 hours to overnight before serving.

Nutrition's Fact: Calories 268, Carbohydrates 24g, Protein 33g, Fat 3g

Fluffy Keto Pancakes

Preparation Time: *20 Minutes Yield: 1 Serving*

Ingredients

- 1 cup almond flour
- 1/4 cup coconut flour
- Two tablespoons low-calorie natural sweetener
- One teaspoon salt
- One teaspoon baking powder
- 1/2 teaspoon ground cinnamon (optional)
- Six eggs, at room temperature
- 1 or 4 cups heavy whipping cream
- Two tablespoons butter, melted
- One teaspoon vanilla extract

Directions

- Mix the almond flour, coconut flour, sweetener, salt, baking powder, and cinnamon in a bowl. Whisk in butter, eggs, heavy cream, and vanilla extract gently until the batter is just blended.
- Heat a lightly oiled skillet over medium-high temperature. Drop the batter by large the spoonfuls onto the grill and cook it until bubbles form and the edges are correctly dry for 4 to 5 minutes. Flip and cook it until browned on the other side, 4 to 5 minutes. Repeat with the remaining batter.

Nutrition's Fact: Calories 265, Carbohydrates 22g, Protein 29g, Fat 5g

Roasted Brussels Sprouts

Preparation Time: *20 Minutes Yield: 1 Serving*

Ingredients

- Two tablespoons olive oil
- One onion, chopped
- 1 pound whole Brussels sprouts
- One teaspoon salt
- 1/2 teaspoon ground black pepper
- 1/2 cup vegetable broth

Directions

- Turn on a pressure cooker and select the Saute function. Heat the olive oil and cook onion until it translucent, about 5 minutes. Add Brussels sprouts and cook it for 2 minutes more. Sprinkle appropriately with salt and pepper; then pour vegetable broth over Brussels sprouts.
- Close and lock the lid. Select the high pressure according to the manufacturer's instructions; set the timer for 5 minutes. Allow 15 to 16 minutes for pressure to build.   Release the cooker's influence carefully using the quick-release method according to the manufacturer's instructions, about 5 minutes. Unlock and remove the lid.

Nutrition's Fact: Calories 264, Carbohydrates 20g, Protein 35g, Fat 4g

Low-Carb Bacon Cheeseburger Casserole

Preparation Time: *20 Minutes Yield: 1 Serving*

Ingredients

- 2 pounds ground beef
- Two cloves garlic, minced
- 1/2 teaspoon onion powder
- 1 pound bacon, cut into small pieces
- Eight eggs
- 1 cup heavy whipping cream
- 1/2 teaspoon salt
- 1/4 teaspoon ground black pepper
- 1 (12 ounces) package shredded Cheddar cheese, divided

Directions

- First, preheat the oven carefully to 350 degrees F.
- Heat a large skillet over medium-high temperature. Cook and stir the beef with garlic and onion powder until it browned and crumbly, 10 to 12 minutes. Drain and discard grease.
- Spread the beef onto the bottom of a 9x13-inch casserole pan. Stir it in bacon pieces.
- Whisk salt, eggs, heavy cream, and pepper in a bowl until well combined. Stir it in 8 ounces Cheddar cheese.
- Pour the egg mix over the beef and bacon. Top it with the remaining 4 ounces of cheese.
- Bake it properly in the preheated oven until golden brown on top, 30 to 35 minutes.

Nutrition's Fact: Calories 261, Carbohydrates 19g, Protein 31g, Fat 3g

Keto Shrimp Scampi with Broccoli Noodles

Preparation Time: *20 Minutes Yield: 1 Serving*

Ingredients

- Two large heads of broccoli with long stems
- Two tablespoons olive oil, divided
- salt and ground black pepper to taste
- Two cloves garlic, minced
- 1 pound raw shrimp, peeled and deveined
- Two tablespoons dry white wine
- Two tablespoons lemon juice
- Two tablespoons butter
- One tablespoon minced fresh basil
- One tablespoon chopped fresh chives
- ½ teaspoon crushed red pepper

Directions

- Cut off the broccoli florets and save them for another use. Cut the woody ends off the stems. Shave the large knots off the branches using a vegetable peeler to be as uniform as possible. Cut it into noodles using the smallest blade on a spiralizer.
- Heat the one tablespoon olive oil in a large skillet over medium-high temperature. Add salt, broccoli noodles, and pepper; toss for 5 minutes. Remove it from heat properly and set it aside.
- Warm the remaining olive oil and garlic in a separate skillet over medium heat. Cook it for 5 minutes, add shrimp and cook until opaque, about 3 minutes per side — transfer shrimp to a bowl.

- Add butter, basil, chives, wine, lemon juice, and red pepper to the skillet. Whisk over medium temperature for 5 minutes. Return the shrimp to the skillet and toss to coat.
- Spoon the broccoli noodles into four serving bowls. Top with shrimp mixture.

Nutrition's Fact: Calories 215, Carbohydrates 25g, Protein 36g, Fat 2g

Rebekah's Keto Egg Casserole

Preparation Time: *20 Minutes Yield: 1 Serving*

Ingredients

- 1 (8 ounces) package breakfast sausage
- 12 eggs
- 1 (8 ounces) package shredded Cheddar cheese
- 3/4 cup heavy whipping cream
- One tablespoon minced onion
- Two teaspoons dry mustard
- One teaspoon dried oregano
- salt and ground black pepper to taste

Directions

- First, preheat the oven properly to 350 degrees F.
- Heat a large skillet over medium-high temperature. Cook the sausage, breaking it alone with a wooden spoon until browned and crumbly, 8 to 9 minutes. Spread it over the bottom of a 9x13-inch casserole dish.
- Mix cream, onion, mustard, oregano, salt, eggs, Cheddar cheese, and pepper together in a bowl. Pour the mix over the sausage.
- Bake it in the preheated oven until firm and cooked for 30 to 40 minutes.

Nutrition's Fact: Calories 260, Carbohydrates 18g, Protein 30g, Fat 2g

Easy Keto Beef Tacos

Preparation Time: *20 Minutes Yield: 1 Serving*

Ingredients

- 2 cups shredded Cheddar cheese
- 1 pound ground beef
- 1/2 package taco seasoning mix
- 1/2 teaspoon salt
- 1/4 teaspoon ground black pepper
- One avocado, diced
- 1 cup shredded lettuce
- 1/2 cup shredded Cheddar cheese
- 1/2 cup tomatoes, diced

Directions

- Preheat the oven properly to 350 degrees F. Line the two baking sheets with parchment paper or a silicone mat.
- Spread the Cheddar cheese into four 6-inch circles, placed them 2 inches apart.
- Bake it in the preheated oven until cheese melts and is lightly brown, 6 to 8 minutes.
- Cold it for 5 minutes before lifting with a spatula. Place over the wooden spoon handle wrapped in aluminum foil supported over 2 cups. Let taco shells cool thoroughly, about 10 minutes.
- Then cook the beef of a skillet over average-high temperature until browned, often stirring to separate meat, about 8 minutes. Season it properly with taco seasoning, salt, and pepper; cook it for 5 minutes more.
- Divide beef mixture among cheese taco shells. Top with avocado, lettuce, Cheddar cheese, and tomatoes.

Oven-Baked Bacon

Preparation Time: *20 Minutes Yield: 1 Serving*

Ingredients

- 1 (16 ounces) package bacon

Directions

- First, preheat the oven carefully to 350 degrees F. Line a baking sheet with parchment paper.
- Put the bacon slices one next to the other on the prepared baking sheet.
- Bake it in the preheated oven properly for 15 to 20 minutes. Remove from the oven. Flip bacon slices with kitchen tongs and return to the range. Bake it until crispy, 15 to 20 minutes more. Thinner slices will need less time, about 20 minutes total. Drain it properly on a plate lined with paper towels.

Nutrition's Fact: Calories 263, Carbohydrates 19g, Protein 33g, Fat 1g

Easy Keto Korean Beef with Cauli Rice

Preparation Time: *20 Minutes Yield: 1 Serving*

Ingredients

- Two teaspoons sesame oil
- 1 pound lean ground beef
- Three cloves garlic, minced
- 1/4 cup soy sauce
- One tablespoon coconut sugar
- 1/4 teaspoon ground ginger
- 1/4 teaspoon ground black pepper
- 2 cups cauliflower rice
- Two tablespoons chopped green onions
- One tablespoon sesame seeds

Directions

- Heat the sesame oil carefully in a medium skillet over medium-high temperature. Cook it and stir the ground beef and garlic in the hot skillet until browned and crumbly, 5 to 7 minutes.
- Combine soy sauce, coconut sugar, ginger, and black pepper in a bowl; whisk until well combined. Pour over ground beef; simmer until the sauce thickens, about 3 minutes.
- Serve over cauliflower rice. Sprinkle with green onions and sesame seeds.

Nutrition's Fact: Calories 262, Carbohydrates 21g, Protein 34g, Fat 4g

Keto Creme Brulee

Preparation Time: *20 Minutes Yield: 1 Serving*

Ingredients

- Four egg yolks
- One teaspoon vanilla extract
- 2 cups heavy whipping cream
- Five tablespoons low-calorie natural sweetener

Directions

- Preheat the oven properly to 325 degrees F.
- Whisk the vanilla extract and egg yolks in a bowl.
- Pour the heavy whipping cream and one tablespoon sweetener into a saucepan over medium heat. Whisk it continually until it starts to simmer. Remove from heat; add yolk mixture slowly, frequently whisking, until well mixed. Divide it evenly between 4 ramekins and place them in a glass baking dish; pour in sufficient boiling water to come 1 inch up the ramekins' sides.
- Bake it in the preheated oven on the middle rack until set, about 30 minutes.
- Sprinkle one tablespoon sweetener over per creme brulee. Use a culinary torch to warm sweetener until melted and golden.

Nutrition's Fact: Calories 264, Carbohydrates 22g, Protein 31g, Fat 6g

Tuscan Pork Tenderloin

Preparation Time: *20 Minutes Yield: 1 Serving*

Ingredients

- Four teaspoons garlic, minced
- Two teaspoons dried rosemary
- Two teaspoons dried oregano
- One teaspoon salt
- One teaspoon ground black pepper
- 4 pounds pork tenderloin

Directions

- Preheat the oven properly to 425 degrees F.
- Combine oregano, salt, garlic, rosemary, and pepper in a bowl. Then rub the spice mix properly all over the pork tenderloin — put it in a baking dish.
- Bake it in the preheated oven until pork is slightly pink in the center, 20 to 30 minutes. An instant-read thermometer inserted into the middle should read at least 140 degrees F. Separate it from the oven and let it properly stand for 10 minutes before slicing.

Nutrition's Fact: Calories 268, Carbohydrates 24g, Protein 33g, Fat 3g

Ketogenic Bread

Preparation Time: *20 Minutes Yield: 1 Serving*

Ingredients

- Seven eggs
- 1/2 cup butter, melted
- Two tablespoons coconut oil
- 2 cups almond flour
- One teaspoon baking powder
- 1/2 teaspoon xanthan gum
- 1/2 teaspoon salt

Directions

- First, preheat the oven carefully to 350 degrees F. Line a loaf pan with parchment paper.
- Then beat the eggs properly in a bowl using an electric mixer on high until frothy, 1 to 2 minutes. Combine butter and coconut oil; continue beating until smooth. Mix xanthan gum, almond flour, baking powder, and salt into egg dough until dough is appropriately combined and very thick; transfer it to the prepared loaf pan.
- Bake it in the preheated oven until a skewer entered in the center comes out clean, about 40 minutes.

Nutrition's Fact: Calories 265, Carbohydrates 22g, Protein 29g, Fat 5g

Low-Carb Pumpkin Cheesecake Bars

Preparation Time: *20 Minutes Yield: 1 Serving*

Ingredients

- cooking spray
- 1 (8 ounces) package cream cheese, softened
- 15 ounces pumpkin puree
- Five eggs
- 1 cup granular sucralose sweetener
- One teaspoon pumpkin pie spice
- One teaspoon ground cinnamon
- One teaspoon vanilla extract

Directions

- Preheat the oven carefully to 350 degrees F. Spray an 8-inch glass baking dish with cooking spray.
- Put the cream cheese smoothly in the bowl of a stand mixer fitted with the paddle attachment; beat on high speed until smooth. Add sweetener, pumpkin pie spice, cinnamon, pumpkin puree, eggs, and vanilla extract. Beat well. Pour batter into the prepared dish.
- Then bake it properly in the preheated oven until the center has set, about 40 minutes. Cool it to room temperature before serving, or serve cold.

Nutrition's Fact: Calories 264, Carbohydrates 20g, Protein 35g, Fat 4g

Chewy Keto Chocolate Cookies

Preparation Time: *20 Minutes Yield: 1 Serving*

Ingredients

- 1 1/2 cups almond butter
- Two eggs
- 1/2 cup low-calorie natural sweetener
- 1/3 cup unsweetened cocoa powder, sifted
- One teaspoon sugar-free vanilla extract
- One pinch salt

Directions

- Preheat the oven properly to 350 degrees F. Line a baking sheet correctly with parchment paper.
- Combine cocoa powder, vanilla extract, almond butter, eggs, sweetener, salt in the bowl of a food processor; pulse until a dough forms.
- Roll the dough into 1-inch balls. Put it carefully on the prepared baking sheet and press down twice with a fork in a criss-cross pattern.
- Bake it in the preheated oven until the edges are firm, about 12 minutes. Cool it on the baking sheet for 5 minutes before removing it to a wire rack to cool completely.

Nutrition's Fact: Calories 261, Carbohydrates 19g, Protein 31g, Fat 3g

Keto Peanut Butter Cookies

Preparation Time: *20 Minutes Yield: 1 Serving*

Ingredients

- 1 cup peanut butter
- 1/2 cup low-calorie natural sweetener
- One egg
- One teaspoon sugar-free vanilla extract

Directions

- Preheat oven properly to 350 degrees F. Line a baking sheet with parchment paper.
- Combine egg, peanut butter, sweetener, and vanilla extract in a bowl; mix well until a dough has formed.
- Roll the dough into 1-inch balls. Place it on the cooked baking sheet and press down twice with a fork in a criss-cross pattern.
- Bake it in the preheated oven properly until the edges are golden, 12 to 15 minutes. Freeze it entirely on the baking sheet for 10 minutes before transferring it to a wire rack to cool completely.

Nutrition's Fact: Calories 215, Carbohydrates 25g, Protein 36g, Fat 2g

Cheesy Keto Biscuits

Preparation Time: *20 Minutes Yield: 1 Serving*

Ingredients

- 2 cups almond flour
- One tablespoon baking powder
- 2 1/2 cups shredded Cheddar cheese
- Four eggs
- 1/4 cup half-and-half

Directions

- Preheat the oven carefully to 350 degrees F. Line a baking sheet with parchment paper.
- Combine the almond flour and baking powder properly in a large bowl. Stir in Cheddar cheese by hand. Build a small well in the middle of the pan; combine eggs and half-and-half to the center. Use a fork, spoon to blend in the flour dough until a sticky batter forms.
- Drop nine portions of batter onto the prepared baking sheet.
- Bake it properly in the preheated oven until golden, about 20 minutes.

Nutrition's Fact: Calories 260, Carbohydrates 18g, Protein 30g, Fat 2g

Lemon Rotisserie Chicken

Preparation Time: *20 Minutes Yield: 1 Serving*

Ingredients

- 1 (2.5 pounds) whole chicken
- One lemon, cut into four wedges
- Two tablespoons olive oil
- 1 1/2 teaspoons salt
- One teaspoon garlic powder
- One teaspoon paprika
- 1/2 teaspoon ground black pepper
- 1 cup chicken broth

Directions

- Rinse chicken and pat dry. Insert lemon wedges inside the cavity.
- Turn it on a multi-functional pressure cooker and select Saute function. Mix paprika, olive oil, salt, garlic powder, and pepper in a bowl. Rub top part of chicken with 1 or 2 of the spice mix. Place the chicken, breast the side down, and cook it until crispy, 5 to 9 minutes.
- Rub the resting spice dough on the bottom side of the chicken. Flip the chicken over with tongs and cook for 5 minutes more.
- Remove chicken from the pot. Place the trivet inside the pan, place the chicken back in the bowl, breast the side down it on the trivet, and pour it in chicken broth. Close and secure the lid. Select the high pressure according to the manufacturer's instructions; set the timer for 20 minutes. Allow 10 to 15 minutes for the weight to build. Release weight properly using

the natural-release system according to the manufacturer's instructions, 15 to 45 minutes.

Nutrition's Fact: Calories 261, Carbohydrates 17g, Protein 31g, Fat 5g

Quick and Easy Parmesan Zucchini Fries

Preparation Time: *20 Minutes Yield: 1 Serving*

Ingredients

- cooking spray
- Two eggs
- 3/4 cup grated Parmesan cheese
- One tablespoon dried mixed herbs
- 1 1/2 teaspoons garlic powder
- One teaspoon paprika
- 1 or 2 teaspoon ground black pepper
- 2 pounds zucchinis

Directions

- Preheat the oven carefully to 425 degrees F. Line a baking sheet with aluminum foil and properly spray it with cooking spray.
- Whisk the eggs in a shallow bowl. Combine the paprika, Parmesan cheese, mixed herbs, garlic powder, and pepper in a separate shallow bowl; mix properly.
- Dip zucchini fries into beaten eggs in batches; shake it to remove excess, and roll in Parmesan mix until completely coated. Place it on the cooked baking sheet.
- Bake it in the preheated oven, turning once, until it was golden and crispy, 30 to 35 minutes.

Nutrition's Fact: Calories 263, Carbohydrates 19g, Protein 33g, Fat 1g

Quick Keto Chocolate Mousse

Preparation Time: *20 Minutes Yield: 1 Serving*

Ingredients

- 3 ounces cream cheese, softened
- 1/2 cup heavy cream
- One teaspoon vanilla extract
- 1/4 cup powdered zero-calorie sweetener
- Two tablespoons cocoa powder
- One pinch salt

Directions

- Place the cream cheese spontaneously in a medium bowl and beat using an electric mixer until light and fluffy. Turn the mixer properly to low speed and slowly add heavy cream and vanilla extract. Add sweetener, cocoa powder, and salt, mixing it until adequately incorporated. Turn the mixer to high, and mix it until light and fluffy, 5 minutes more. Serve it immediately, or refrigerate for later.

Nutrition's Fact: Calories 262, Carbohydrates 21g, Protein 34g, Fat 4g

Baked Lemon-Butter Chicken Thighs

Preparation Time: *20 Minutes Yield: 1 Serving*

Ingredients

- Four tablespoons butter, divided
- Four cloves garlic
- Two tablespoons lemon juice
- 1/4 teaspoon onion powder
- 4 (8 ounces) skin-on, bone-in chicken thighs
- salt and ground black pepper to taste
- Two tablespoons fresh parsley, chopped

Directions

- Preheat the oven carefully to 375 degrees F.
- Place three tablespoons butter in a microwave-safe bowl and heat in a microwave oven until melted, 5 minutes. Smash the garlic cloves properly with the side of a chef's knife and add garlic to the hot butter. Stir in lemon juice and onion powder. Set it aside.
- Sprinkle all sides of chicken thighs properly with salt and pepper. Heat the remaining one tablespoon butter properly in a medium-sized oven-safe skillet over medium-high heat. Brown the chicken, skin-side down, for 10 minutes, flip the chicken over, and brush the skin with the lemon-butter dough. Pour the remaining butter mixture into a skillet and separate it from heat.
- Bake it in the preheated oven until chicken is no longer pink at the bone and the juices run clear for about 35 minutes. An instant-read thermometer entered near the bone should read 160 degrees F. Brush skin every 15 minutes with pan juices.

- Transfer the skillet from the oven and place chicken on a serving platter. Drizzle chicken with pan juices and garnish with parsley.

Nutrition's Fact: Calories 264, Carbohydrates 22g, Protein 31g, Fat 6g

Keto Cauliflower Hash Browns

Ingredients

- 3 cups grated cauliflower
- 1 cup shredded Cheddar cheese
- One large egg
- 1/4 cup real bacon bits
- One tablespoon diced chives
- 1/2 teaspoon salt
- 1/8 teaspoon ground black pepper
- One pinch of cayenne pepper (optional)
- cooking spray

Directions

- Preheat the oven carefully to 400 degrees F.
- Place the grated cauliflower in a microwave-safe bowl. Cook it on high for 2 minutes, let cool for 10 minutes.
- Wring the cauliflower in a clean dish towel, squeezing out as much moisture as possible. Transfer the cauliflower to a large mixing bowl adds bacon bits, chives, salt, pepper, Cheddar cheese, egg, and cayenne. Mix it properly.
- Spray a baking sheet with cooking spray. Divide the cauliflower mix into six equal portions, making assured to leave space between per one. Flatten with your hands and shape it into ovals.
- Bake it in the preheated oven until appropriately browned, about 15 minutes. Turn the broiler on low and then broil until crispy, about 10 minutes. Let it cool for 5 minutes to firm up.

Nutrition's Fact: Calories 268, Carbohydrates 24g, Protein 33g, Fat 3g

Keto Cinnamon Granola

Preparation Time: *20 Minutes Yield: 1 Serving*

Ingredients

- 1/2 cup coarsely chopped walnuts
- 1/2 cup coarsely chopped pecans
- 1/2 cup unsweetened shredded coconut
- 1/3 cup sliced almonds
- One teaspoon ground cinnamon
- Two teaspoons granulated erythritol sweetener
- Two tablespoons butter, melted

Directions

- Preheat oven carefully to 375 degrees F.
- Mix the coconut, walnuts, pecans, and almonds in a bowl.
- Stir cinnamon, Erythritol, and Sucralose into softened butter properly. Then pour it over the nut mixture and stir it to coat — spread the granola in a single layer on a baking sheet.
- Bake it in the preheated oven until crunchy, 15 minutes. Please remove it from the oven, stir it, and allow it to cool.

Nutrition's Fact: Calories 265, Carbohydrates 22g, Protein 29g, Fat 5g

Chicken Tikka Masala

Preparation Time: *20 Minutes Yield: 1 Serving*

Ingredients

- 1 pound boneless chicken breasts
- One cup plain yogurt
- One tablespoon garam masala
- One tablespoon lemon juice
- One teaspoon cayenne pepper
- One pinch ground ginger
- 1 (15 ounces) can tomato sauce
- Four cloves garlic, minced
- 1 1/2 tablespoons garam masala
- One teaspoon paprika
- 1/2 teaspoon ground turmeric
- 1/2 teaspoon salt
- 1 cup heavy cream

Directions

- Combine the lemon juice, cayenne pepper, chicken, yogurt, garam masala, ginger in a bowl; toss until fully coated. Cover and refrigerate it for 60 min.
- Turn on a pressure cooker and select Saute function. Add chicken with marinade; cook until tender, occasionally stirring, about 10 minutes.
- Place garam masala, paprika, turmeric, tomato sauce, garlic, and salt in the pot; stir until properly mixed. Close and lock the lid. Select high pressure according to the manufacturer's directions; set the timer for 15 minutes. Provide 10 to 15 minutes for pressure to build.

- Release the pressure correctly using the quick-release system according to the manufacturer's commands, about 10 minutes. Separate lid and select the Saute function. Pour it in cream; stir it well. Simmer it until the sauce has thickened, about 5 minutes.

Nutrition's Fact: Calories 264, Carbohydrates 20g, Protein 35g, Fat 4g

Grain-Free Butter Bread

Preparation Time: *20 Minutes Yield: 1 Serving*

Ingredients

- Six eggs
- 1 or 2 cups finely ground almond flour
- One teaspoon fine salt
- Two teaspoons baking powder
- 1/4 cup melted butter
- 1/8 teaspoon cream of tartar

Directions

- Separate the eggs. Crack per egg into your hand and let the whites properly run into a bowl. Place the yolks in a 2nd bowl.
- Preheat the oven to 376 degrees F. Butter a loaf pan and then line the bottom with parchment paper.
- Put the almond flour in a food processor. Add baking powder, salt, and egg yolks. Pour it in melted butter. Then pulse, scraping down the sides once or twice until the dough comes together.
- Sprinkle the cream of tartar into the egg whites. Whisk until soft peaks form. Transfer about 1 or 3 of the mixture into the food processor. Pulse on and off, scraping the dough down with a spatula as required, until well blended. Scrape mix into the bowl with the egg whites. Fold together until adequately mixed but still airy. Pour the batter carefully into the prepared loaf pan.
- Then bake it in the preheated oven until golden brown and a toothpick inserted into the center comes out clean, about 35 minutes.

- Run a thin knife along with the edge bread and let rest for 10 minutes. Turn the dough out onto a wire rack and cool to room temperature before slicing.

Nutrition's Fact: Calories 261, Carbohydrates 19g, Protein 31g, Fat 3g

Steamed Artichokes

Preparation Time: *20 Minutes Yield: 1 Serving*

Ingredients

- 1 cup of water
- Two cloves garlic
- One bay leaf
- 1/2 teaspoon salt
- Four artichokes
- Two tablespoons lemon juice

Directions

- Combine the bay leaf, water, garlic, and salt inside a multi-functional pressure cooker. Place the steamer in the pot. Combine artichokes, trimmed top facing up, drizzle it with lemon juice. Close it and lock the lid. Select the high pressure according to the manufacturer's directions; set the timer for 10 minutes. Release 10 minutes for pressure to build.
- Release pressure carefully using the quick-release system according to the manufacturer's directions, about 5 minutes. Unlock and remove the lid.
- Cool it until easily handled. Pull it off outer petals one at a time. Pull through teeth to separate the soft portion of the leaf. Discard remaining petal. Spoon out a fuzzy center near the stem and then discard. Eat the bottom whole or cut it into pieces.

Nutrition's Fact: Calories 215, Carbohydrates 25g, Protein 36g, Fat 2g

Low-Carb Almond Coconut Sandies

Preparation Time: *20 Minutes Yield: 1 Serving*

Ingredients

- 1 cup unsweetened coconut
- 1 cup almond meal
- 1/3 cup coconut oil, melted
- One egg white
- Two tablespoons water
- One tablespoon vanilla extract
- One teaspoon Himalayan sea salt
- 1 or 3 teaspoon stevia powder

Directions

- Preheat the oven carefully to 325 degrees F. Line a baking sheet with parchment paper.
- Combine coconut oil, egg white, water, vanilla extract, Himalayan sea salt, coconut, almond meal, and stevia powder in a large bowl. Let sit until coconut melts, about 10 minutes. Roll into generous tablespoon-sized balls; place on a baking sheet. Flatten it gently with a fork to prevent edges from crumbling.
- Bake it in the preheated oven properly until the edges are golden, 13 to 15 minutes. Cool it on the baking sheet for 5 minutes before removing it to a wire rack to cool completely.

Nutrition's Fact: Calories 260, Carbohydrates 18g, Protein 30g, Fat 2g

Best Keto Bread

Preparation Time: *20 Minutes Yield: 1 Serving*

Ingredients

- cooking spray
- Seven eggs, at room temperature
- 1/2 cup butter, melted and cooled
- Two tablespoons olive oil
- 2 cups blanched almond flour
- One teaspoon baking powder
- 1/2 teaspoon xanthan gum
- 1/2 teaspoon sea salt

Directions

- First, preheat the oven carefully to 350 degrees F or 175 degrees C. Then, grease a silicone loaf pan with cooking spray.
- Whisk the eggs properly in a bowl until soft and creamy, about 5 minutes. Add the softened butter and olive oil; mix until well combined.
- Combine the xanthan gum, almond flour, baking powder, and salt in a separate bowl; stir well. Combine slowly to the egg mixture, mixing properly until a thick batter has formed.
- Pour the batter properly into the prepared pan and soften the top with a spatula.
- Bake it in the preheated oven until a toothpick inserted into the center comes out clean, about 45 minutes.

Nutrition's Fact: Calories 261, Carbohydrates 17g, Protein 31g, Fat 5g

Keto Broccoli Cheddar Soup

Preparation Time: *20 Minutes Yield: 1 Serving*

Ingredients

- One teaspoon butter
- Three cloves garlic, minced
- 2 ½ cups vegetable broth
- 3 cups chopped broccoli
- 1 cup heavy whipping cream
- 3 cups shredded Cheddar cheese
- Two slices bacon, chopped and cooked
- salt and ground black pepper to taste

Directions

- Melt the butter properly in a saucepan over medium temperature. Cook garlic until tender, about 2 minutes. Add vegetable broth, heavy cream, and broccoli. Take to a boil; simmer it until broccoli is tender, about 15 minutes.
- Add Cheddar cheese gradually, continually stirring, until completely melted. Stir it in the bacon pieces — season it with salt and pepper.

Nutrition's Fact: Calories 263, Carbohydrates 19g, Protein 33g, Fat 1g

Keto Margarita

Preparation Time: *20 Minutes Yield: 1 Serving*

Ingredients

- 3 cups ice
- Two fluid ounces of tequila
- One fluid ounce lime juice
- 1 or 2 teaspoons low-calorie natural sweetener
- One tablespoon coarse salt
- Two lime wedges
- One pint-sized Mason jar
- Two fluid ounces orange-flavored sparkling water

Directions

- Fill a shaker half-full with ice. Add lime juice, tequila, and sweetener to the shaker. Seal it and shake quickly until the outside is frosted, 10 to 15 seconds.
- Place the salt on a plate. Then run the one lime wedge along the rim of the Mason jar. Press the pot down into the salt. Fill the jar with ice cubes.
- Strain margarita into the jar. Top with sparkling water and stir. Garnish with a remaining lime wedge.

Nutrition's Fact: Calories 262, Carbohydrates 21g, Protein 34g, Fat 4g

Keto Open-Faced Chicken Cordon Bleu

Preparation Time: *20 Minutes Yield: 1 Serving*

Ingredients

- 1 pound chicken cutlets
- salt and freshly ground black pepper
- Two eggs
- One teaspoon Dijon mustard
- 2/3 cup almond flour
- 1/3 cup freshly grated Parmesan cheese
- 1/2 teaspoon garlic powder
- 1/4 cup avocado oil
- 1/4 pound shaved deli ham
- 1 cup shredded Swiss cheese

Directions

- Preheat the oven carefully to 375 degrees F. Season the chicken cutlets with salt and pepper; set aside.
- Whisk the eggs and Dijon mustard properly together in a shallow bowl. Then combine the Parmesan cheese, almond flour, and garlic powder in a separate shallow bowl. Dip chicken cutlets into the egg mix, letting excess drip off. Dredge it with almond flour mixture, then set it on a plate.
- Warm the oil spontaneously in a skillet over medium-high temperature. Add chicken cutlets and cook it until golden brown, 5 minutes. Flip it over and cook it until chicken is no longer pink inside and the juices are running clear, 5 minutes also.
- Place the chicken cutlets carefully on a baking sheet. Top with slices of ham and cover it with shredded Swiss cheese.

- Bake it in the preheated oven until cheese has melted, 4 to 5 minutes. Serve immediately.

 Calories 264, Carbohydrates 22g, Protein 31g, Fat 6g

Keto Berry-Pecan Cheesecake Bars

Preparation Time: *20 Minutes Yield: 1 Serving*

Ingredients

- 1 cup pecans
- One teaspoon stevia-erythritol sweetener
- One teaspoon cinnamon
- 1/4 teaspoon ground nutmeg
- Two tablespoons melted butter
- One egg
- 12 ounces cream cheese
- 1/2 cup stevia-erythritol sweetener
- 1/4 cup sour cream
- 1/2 teaspoon vanilla extract
- 1/4 cup unsweetened almond milk
- One tablespoon melted butter
- One cup of frozen mixed berries
- One tablespoon stevia-erythritol sweetener

Directions

- Preheat the oven carefully to 350 degrees F.
- Combine pecans into a food processor and chop them very finely. Add cinnamon, sweetener, and nutmeg and process for a few more seconds. Pour the dough into a bowl and add melted butter. Stir it together, and then press the crust in the mixture into the bottom of a divided brownie pan with the divider separated.
- Beat the egg until fluffy in a large bowl with an electric mixer. Mix it in cream cheese 1 ounce at a time. Then beat the mixture until cream cheese is smooth. Add vanilla extract, sweetener,

sour cream, and almond milk. Beat together until the filling is soft. Then stir it in melted butter. Pour the mixture properly over the crust in the brownie pan. Insert divider into the pan.

- Bake it smoothly in the preheated oven for about 40 minutes.
- Meanwhile, heat a small pot over medium temperature. Combine mixed berries and sweeteners and take to a simmer, about 5 minutes. Stir seeds and crush some with a spoon so that a liquid starts to form — Cook it for about 10 minutes more.
- Allow the cheesecake bars to cool in the brownie pan, about 1 hour. Pour berry sauce on top of bars.

Nutrition's Fact: Calories 268, Carbohydrates 24g, Protein 33g, Fat 3g

Keto Tuna Salad

Preparation Time: *20 Minutes Yield: 1 Serving*

Ingredients

- 2 (6 ounces) cans of water-packed tuna
- 2 (6 ounce) cans olive oil-packed tuna
- 3/4 cup reduced-fat olive oil mayonnaise
- Two stalks celery, chopped
- 1/2 lime, juiced
- 1/4 red onion, chopped
- Two tablespoons mustard
- salt and ground black pepper to taste

Directions

- Combine mayonnaise, red onion, mustard, salt, celery, lime juice, water-packed tuna, oil-packed tuna, and pepper in a bowl. Stir well.

Nutrition's Fact: Calories 265, Carbohydrates 22g, Protein 29g, Fat 5g

Peanut Butter Chocolate Cookies

Preparation Time: *20 Minutes Yield: 1 Serving*

Ingredients

- One cup creamy peanut butter
- One egg
- 1/4 cup stevia sweetener
- Two tablespoons unsweetened cocoa powder
- One tablespoon vanilla extract

Directions

- Preheat oven carefully to 350 degrees F (175 degrees C).
- Combine peanut butter, egg, stevia sweetener, cocoa powder, and vanilla extract with a mixer or food processor. Roll dough into 1-inch balls places 1 to 2 inches apart on an ungreased baking sheet. Flatten balls with a fork.
- Bake it in the preheated oven until edges have set, about 10 minutes. Let it freeze on the baking sheet for 20 minutes.
- Line a tray with waxed paper. Transfer the cookies to the dish until frozen to room heat, about 20 minutes, then refrigerate for 25 minutes.

Nutrition's Fact: Calories 264, Carbohydrates 20g, Protein 35g, Fat 4g

Keto Chicken Cordon Bleu Meatballs

Preparation Time: *20 Minutes Yield: 1 Serving*

Ingredients

- 1 pound ground chicken
- 1/3 cup blanched almond flour
- 1/2 teaspoon salt
- 1/2 teaspoon garlic powder
- 1/2 teaspoon onion powder
- One egg, lightly beaten
- 6 ounces ham steak
- One tablespoon olive oil
- One tablespoon butter
- 3/4 cup chicken broth
- One teaspoon Dijon mustard
- 1/2 cup heavy cream
- 1 cup shredded Swiss cheese
- One pinch cracked black pepper to taste
- Two tablespoons minced fresh parsley (optional)

Directions

- Combine almond flour, salt, garlic powder, chicken, onion powder, and egg in a bowl. Form a little portion of chicken mix into one or 2-inch ball around a cube of ham and place onto a plate. Repeat with the remaining chicken mixture and pork, making 20 meatballs total.
- Warm the olive oil in a skillet over medium-high temperature. Brown meatballs for 5 minutes, turn and cook it an additional 3 to 4 minutes. Transfer meatballs onto a clean plate.

- Return skillet to medium temperature and melt the butter. Whisk it in chicken broth and Dijon mustard and bring to a simmer for 5 minutes. Stir it in heavy cream and whisk until sauce begins to simmer. Whisk it in Swiss cheese until fully melted. Return meatballs to skillet and simmer it until the sauce has slightly thickened, 5 minutes. Season it with cracked black pepper and parsley serve it immediately. The sauce will further thicken upon cooling.

Nutrition's Fact: Calories 261, Carbohydrates 19g, Protein 31g, Fat 3g

Chocolate Fat Bomb

Preparation Time: *20 Minutes Yield: 1 Serving*

Ingredients

- 1 (8 ounces) package cream cheese
- 3 or 4 cups of coconut oil
- 1.4 ounces chocolate pudding mix

Directions

- Blend the coconut oil, cream cheese, and chocolate pudding mix in a bowl using an electric mixer until soft.
- Scoop it into mounds or place it in a mold to form. Cover it adequately with plastic wrap and then refrigerate it until thickened, about 25 minutes.

Nutrition's Fact: Calories 215, Carbohydrates 25g, Protein 36g, Fat 2g

Keto Strawberry Ice Cream

Preparation Time: *20 Minutes Yield: 1 Serving*

Ingredients

- Five strawberries, hulled
- 2 1/2 cups heavy whipping cream
- 2/3 cup low-calorie natural sweetener
- 1/2 cup water
- Two teaspoons vanilla extract
- One teaspoon lemon juice
- 1/2 teaspoon vodka
- One pinch salt

Directions

- Place the strawberries carefully in a food processor or blender; puree until smooth.
- Whisk strawberry puree, cream, sweetener, water, vanilla extract, lemon juice, vodka, and salt together in a bowl; pour into an ice cream maker.
- Then prepare the ice cream according to the manufacturer's directions. Transfer to a freezer-safe container and freeze until firm.

Nutrition's Fact: Calories 260, Carbohydrates 18g, Protein 30g, Fat 2g

Keto Sausage Balls

Preparation Time: *20 Minutes Yield: 1 Serving*

Ingredients

- 1 pound spicy ground pork sausage
- 1/2 (8 ounces) package cream cheese, at room temperature
- 1/2 cup shredded sharp Cheddar cheese
- 1/2 cup grated Parmesan cheese
- One tablespoon Dijon mustard
- 1/2 teaspoon garlic powder
- 1/4 teaspoon salt

Directions

- Preheat the oven carefully to 350 degrees F. Line a baking sheet with parchment paper.
- Combine Cheddar cheese, Parmesan cheese, sausage, cream cheese, mustard, garlic powder, and salt in a medium bowl. Mix it gently until just mixed. Roll the heaping tablespoonfuls of the pork mixture into the balls. Place it on the prepared baking sheet.
- Bake it properly in the preheated oven until golden brown, 30 to 35 minutes. Place on a paper towel-lined plate to soak up excess grease. Serve immediately.

Nutrition's Fact: Calories 261, Carbohydrates 17g, Protein 31g, Fat 5g

Keto Recipe With Mushrooms

Preparation Time: *20 Minutes Yield: 1 Serving*

Ingredients

- One small spaghetti squash
- One tablespoon olive oil
- salt and ground black pepper to taste
- Four slices bacon, cut into 1/2-inch pieces
- 1 (4 ounces) package mushrooms, sliced
- One clove garlic, minced
- 2 cups baby spinach
- 1/4 cup sour cream
- Two tablespoons crumbled blue cheese

Directions

- Preheat the oven carefully to 400 degrees F (200 degrees C). Line a baking sheet correctly with aluminum foil.
- Cut the stem off the end of the spaghetti squash applying a sharp knife. Slice the squash in half lengthwise and then scrape out the seeds. Brush the inside smoothly with olive oil and sprinkle it with salt and pepper.
- Bake it in the preheated oven until soft, about 44 minutes. Scrape the cooked flesh out into a bowl and set it aside.
- Place bacon carefully in a medium skillet and cook over medium-high temperature, occasionally turning, until evenly browned 6 to 7 minutes. Drain bacon slices properly on paper towels.
- Combine mushrooms and garlic into the skillet and cook it for 4 to 5 minutes. Add in the cooked bacon and spinach. Stir until the spinach has wilted, 2 to 3 minutes. Combine mushroom

mixture into the bowl of squash. Mix in sour cream, salt, and pepper. Stir until filling is evenly combined.

- Spoon filling back into the squash shells. Sprinkle each half with one tablespoon of blue cheese. Please return to the oven and then bake it until cheese has melted and squash has heated through 4 to 5 minutes.

Nutrition's Fact: Calories 263, Carbohydrates 19g, Protein 33g, Fat 1g

Keto Crack Chicken

Preparation Time: *20 Minutes Yield: 1 Serving*

Ingredients

- 2 pounds skinless, boneless chicken breast
- 1 (8 ounces) package cream cheese
- 1 (1 ounce) package ranch dressing mix
- 1/2 cup water
- Six slices cooked bacon, chopped
- 1 cup Cheddar cheese

Directions

- Combine the chicken and cream cheese in a multi-functional pressure cooker. Sprinkle it with ranch seasoning and add water. Close and lock the lid. Select the high pressure according to the manufacturer's directions; set the timer for 16 minutes. Allow 18 minutes for pressure to build.
- Then release the pressure carefully using the quick-release method according to the manufacturer's instructions, about 5 minutes. Unlock and remove the lid.
- Remove the chicken and then shred using two forks; return chicken to the pot. Select low heat according to the manufacturer's directions. Add Cheddar cheese and bacon. Stir it to combine and warm through 2 to 3 minutes.

Nutrition's Fact: Calories 262, Carbohydrates 21g, Protein 34g, Fat 4g

Keto Avocado Dessert

Preparation Time: *20 Minutes Yield: 1 Serving*

Ingredients

- One ripe avocado - peeled, pitted, and diced
- 1/4 cup heavy whipping cream
- 1/2 teaspoon liquid stevia
- 1/4 teaspoon vanilla extract
- 1/4 teaspoon ground cinnamon

Directions

- Mash the avocado in a bowl. Combine heavy cream, stevia, vanilla, and cinnamon; mix it thoroughly.
- Finally, refrigerate the avocado mixture for 1 hour before serving.

Nutrition's Fact: Calories 264, Carbohydrates 22g, Protein 31g, Fat 6g

Keto NY Cheesecake

Preparation Time: *20 Minutes Yield: 1 Serving*

Ingredients

- 2/3 cup almond meal
- Five tablespoons butter, melted
- 2 (8 ounces) packages of cream cheese
- 3/4 cup low-calorie natural sweetener
- 1/4 cup heavy whipping cream
- Two tablespoons water
- Three eggs
- 1/2 cup sour cream
- Two tablespoons almond flour
- 1 1/2 teaspoons vanilla extract

Directions

- Preheat the oven carefully to 350 degrees F. Line a 12-cup muffin pan with paper liners.
- Mix the almond meal and butter in a bowl. Spoon it into the bottoms of the paper liners; press it down to form a flat crust.
- Stir the cream cheese and sweetener together in a bowl just until smooth. Mix it in whipping cream and water add eggs one at a time, whisking well after each addition. Stir it in sour cream, almond flour, and vanilla extract. Spoon it into paper liners.
- Bake it properly in the preheated oven until the cream cheese mixture is almost set in the center, 20 minutes. Be aware not to overcook.
- Let it cool at room temperature; refrigerate it 8 hours to overnight.

 Calories 268, Carbohydrates 24g, Protein 33g, Fat 3g

Spicy Keto Chicken-and-Cheese Casserole

Preparation Time: *20 Minutes Yield: 1 Serving*

Ingredients

- One teaspoon butter, or as needed
- Four skinless, boneless chicken breasts, cut into chunks
- One teaspoon taco seasoning mix, or to taste
- 1 (8 ounces) jar salsa
- 1/2 cup sour cream
- 4 ounces jalapeno peppers, diced
- 4 ounces shredded Cheddar cheese
- Four green onions, sliced

Directions

- Preheat the oven carefully to 350 degrees F (174 degrees C). Butter a baking pan.
- Heat a pan over medium-high heat. Add the chicken and then saute until no longer pink in the center, and juices run clear for 6 to 8 minutes. Drain excess liquid. Add taco seasoning; toss it to coat — transfer chicken into the prepared baking pan.
- Mix salsa, sour cream, and jalapenos in a bowl and pour it over the chicken.
- Bake it in the preheated oven until hot, about 22 minutes. Please remove it from the oven and cover it with Cheddar cheese. Continue baking properly until the cheese melts, about 10 minutes also.
- Let casserole cool before cutting into pieces and garnishing with green onions.

Nutrition's Fact: Calories 265, Carbohydrates 22g, Protein 29g, Fat 5g

Easy Keto Homemade Tomato Sauce

Preparation Time: *20 Minutes Yield: 1 Serving*

Ingredients

- 1 (28 ounces) can San Marzano-style peeled plum tomatoes
- 1/4 cup extra-virgin olive oil
- One teaspoon garlic powder
- One teaspoon dried basil
- One teaspoon salt
- 1/2 teaspoon dried oregano
- 1/2 teaspoon ground black pepper

Directions

- Place the tomatoes and the olive oil in a blender, then pulse it until smooth. Add basil, salt, oregano, garlic powder, and pepper; mix it until well combined.

Nutrition's Fact: Calories 264, Carbohydrates 20g, Protein 35g, Fat 4g

Best Low-Carb Keto Meatballs

Preparation Time: *20 Minutes Yield: 1 Serving*

Ingredients

- 1 1/2 pounds ground beef
- One egg
- Two tablespoons grated Parmesan cheese
- One tablespoon flaxseed meal
- One teaspoon dried oregano
- salt and ground black pepper to taste
- One tablespoon olive oil
- 1 (14 ounces) can tomato sauce

Directions

- Combine egg, Parmesan cheese, flaxseed, ground beef, oregano, salt, and pepper in a bowl; mix it until thoroughly combined. Roll mixture into golf-ball-size meatballs.
- Heat the olive oil properly in a large skillet over medium temperature. Add the meatballs; cook until browned, about 5 minutes on each side. Pour the tomato sauce over meatballs; simmer for 32 minutes.

Nutrition's Fact: Calories 261, Carbohydrates 19g, Protein 31g, Fat 3g

Sheet Pan Ratatouille

Preparation Time: *20 Minutes Yield: 1 Serving*

Ingredients

- One large eggplant, cut into 1/2-inch cubes
- Two zucchinis, cut into 1/2-inch slices
- Two heirloom tomatoes, cut in wedges
- One white onion, cut into 1/2-inch-thick rounds
- One red bell pepper, cut into 1/2-inch strips
- Four cloves garlic
- Two tablespoons olive oil
- Two tablespoons chopped fresh rosemary
- One teaspoon salt
- 1/2 teaspoon ground black pepper
- One tablespoon balsamic vinegar

Directions

- Preheat the oven carefully to 400 degrees F (200 degrees C). Line a baking sheet with parchment paper.
- Place the tomatoes, onion, bell pepper, eggplant, zucchinis, and garlic in a single layer on the prepared baking sheet. Drizzle it with olive oil, salt, rosemary, and pepper; toss vegetables until well coated.
- Roast in the preheated oven until slightly tender; about 20 minutes. Mix and roast for another 12 minutes. Decrease the temperature properly to 300 degrees F and cook it until vegetables begin to caramelize; about 10 minutes. Drizzle with balsamic vinegar.

Nutrition's Fact: Calories 215, Carbohydrates 25g, Protein 36g, Fat 2g

Keto Raspberry Fudge

Preparation Time: *20 Minutes Yield: 1 Serving*

Ingredients

- 1 cup butter
- 8 ounces cream cheese
- Six tablespoons unsweetened cocoa powder
- 1/3 cup chopped walnuts
- 1/4 cup white sugar substitute
- Two tablespoons heavy cream
- Two teaspoons vanilla extract
- One teaspoon raspberry extract

Directions

- Beat the butter and then cream the cheese together in a large microwave-safe bowl working an electric mixer until smooth it suitably. Add sugar substitute, heavy cream, vanilla extract, cocoa powder, walnuts, and raspberry extract. Stir fudge mixture slowly until well combined.
- Microwave the fudge mix on high, about 25 seconds. Continue blending until smooth. Grease a 9x13 baking pan; spread batter into the pot in 1 soft layer, cover it with plastic wrap, and then refrigerate until set, at least 2 hours. Cut into bars.

Nutrition's Fact: Calories 260, Carbohydrates 18g, Protein 30g, Fat 2g

Cauliflower-Spinach Side Dish

Preparation Time: *20 Minutes Yield: 1 Serving*

Ingredients

- 2 3/4 cups cauliflower florets
- 2 cups spinach leaves
- Two tablespoons butter
- One teaspoon sea salt
- Two spreadable cheese wedges

Directions

- Run the cauliflower carefully through a food processor to prepare 2 cups of cauliflower grounds a bit larger than grits' density.
- Combine butter, cauliflower, spinach, and salt in a large pot over low heat. Cover and cook it until cauliflower is smooth and spinach has wilted for 5 to 7 minutes. Stir it in cheese wedges until the cauliflower and spinach have coated, and no cheese clumps remain.

Nutrition's Fact: Calories 261, Carbohydrates 17g, Protein 31g, Fat 5g

Chocolate-Peanut Butter Keto Cups

Preparation Time: *20 Minutes Yield: 1 Serving*

Ingredients

- 1 cup of coconut oil
- 1/2 cup natural peanut butter
- Two tablespoons heavy cream
- One tablespoon cocoa powder
- One teaspoon liquid stevia
- 1/4 teaspoon vanilla extract
- 1/4 teaspoon kosher salt
- 1 ounce chopped roasted salted peanuts

Directions

- Melt the coconut oil smoothly in a saucepan over low temperature, 5 to 6 minutes. Stir in peanut butter until smooth. Whisk in liquid stevia, vanilla extract, heavy cream, cocoa powder, and salt.
- Pour chocolate-peanut butter mix into 12 silicone muffin molds. Sprinkle the peanuts evenly on the top — place the shapes on a baking sheet.
- Freeze chocolate-peanut butter mix until firm, at least 60 min. Unmold the chocolate-peanut cups and shift to a resealable plastic bag or airtight container.

Nutrition's Fact: Calories 263, Carbohydrates 19g, Protein 33g, Fat 1g

Keto Cheesecake Brownies

Preparation Time: *20 Minutes Yield: 1 Serving*

Ingredients

- 1 cup cream cheese, softened
- 1/4 cup stevia powder
- One egg
- One teaspoon vanilla extract
- 1/2 cup unsalted butter
- 1/2 cup stevia powder
- 1/3 cup cocoa powder
- 1/2 teaspoon salt
- Two eggs
- 1/3 cup almond flour

Directions

- Preheat the oven carefully to 350 degrees F. Line an 8-inch square pan with parchment paper.
- Mix cream cheese and stevia in a bowl using an electric mixer until creamy smooth. Mix in egg and vanilla extract until thoroughly mixed.
- Take a saucepan of water to a simmer. Top pan with a heatproof bowl large enough to stay above the water combine butter, stevia, cocoa powder, and salt in the container. Cook and stir until melted and thoroughly combined, 1 to 3 minutes. Remove from heat and cool until the dish is secured to handle. Whisk it in 1 egg at a time, stirring vigorously, until the dough becomes pudding-like. Add almond flour and continue to whisk the brownie mixture until blended.

- Pour 2 or 3 of the brownie mixture into the bottom of the prepared baking pan. Combine cream cheese mixture. Top with dollops of the remaining brownie mix and use a knife to create a swirled design.
- Bake it in the preheated oven until set but still slightly jiggly, about 25 minutes. Cool before serving.

Nutrition's Fact: Calories 262, Carbohydrates 21g, Protein 34g, Fat 4g

Keto Coconut Lime Bars

Preparation Time: *20 Minutes Yield: 1 Serving*

Ingredients

- 1 cup finely ground almond flour
- 1/4 cup low-calorie natural sweetener
- Two tablespoons coconut flour
- One teaspoon lime zest
- 1/4 teaspoon salt
- Three tablespoons butter softened
- 1 cup lime juice
- 1/2 cup coconut milk
- 1/2 cup low-calorie natural powdered sweetener
- One tablespoon butter
- One teaspoon lime zest
- Five large eggs, beaten
- Two tablespoons unsweetened coconut
- 1/2 tablespoon lime zest

Directions

- Preheat the oven carefully to 350 degrees F (175 degrees C) — grease an 8x8-inch baking dish.
- Mix the almond flour, sweetener, coconut flour, lime zest, and salt in a large bowl. Mix thoroughly. Cut in butter with a fork until mixed, and no lumps remain — press the crust mixture down into the prepared baking dish.
- Bake in the preheated oven until gently browned, 10 to 15 minutes. Set aside.

- Whisk sweetener, butter, lime juice, coconut milk, and zest in a medium saucepan over medium heat. Mix until sweetener has dissolved; do not let boil. Combine beaten eggs slowly, a little at a time, continually whisking until mixture is foamy and airy and starts to thicken, 15 minutes. Remove the filling mixture from heat and spread evenly over the crust.
- Bake in the preheated oven until the filling has set in the center, 10 to 15 minutes.
- Toast the shredded coconut in a skillet over medium temperature until lightly browned, 5 minutes. Sprinkle the coconut and lime zest topping over the bars. Let it cool and refrigerate completely before cutting into bars.

Nutrition's Fact: Calories 264, Carbohydrates 22g, Protein 31g, Fat 6g

Keto Peanut Butter Fudge Fat Bomb

Preparation Time: *20 Minutes Yield: 1 Serving*

Ingredients

- 1 cup unsweetened peanut butter, softened
- 1 cup of coconut oil
- 1/4 cup unsweetened vanilla-flavored almond milk
- Two teaspoons vanilla liquid stevia, or as needed (optional)

Directions

- Line a loaf pan with parchment paper.
- Combine the peanut butter and the coconut oil in a microwave-safe dish. Microwave 25 seconds until lightly melted. Add it to the blender with almond milk and stevia; blend it until well mixed. Pour it into a loaf pan and refrigerate until set, about 2 hours.

Nutrition's Fact: Calories 268, Carbohydrates 24g, Protein 33g, Fat 3g

Keto Crackers

Preparation Time: *20 Minutes Yield: 1 Serving*

Ingredients

- 1/2 cup shredded mozzarella cheese
- 1/3 cup finely ground almond flour
- 1/8 teaspoon garlic powder
- 1/8 teaspoon salt
- One large egg yolk

Directions

- Preheat the oven carefully to 425 degrees F. Line a baking sheet with parchment paper.
- Combine almond flour, garlic powder, mozzarella cheese, and salt in a microwave-safe bowl. Heat in the microwave for 30 seconds.
- Use your hands to knead the mozzarella mixture until thoroughly appropriately mixed. Combine egg yolk and continue kneading until smoothly blended into the mix.
- Lay a slice of parchment paper on a flat surface and place dough on top. Place the second piece of parchment paper on top of the mix. Press down it on the dough with your hands until you are ready for a rolling pin. Roll into a skinny rectangle with flat sides. Gently poke holes in the mixture using a fork to prevent it from boiling while baking. Cut the dough smoothly into 1-inch squares with a knife.
- Lay squares on the served baking sheet, leaving a little space between them
- Bake it properly in the preheated oven for 5 minutes. Remove the baking sheet from the oven and turn the crackers over.

Bake it on the other side until quickly browned and crisp, two more minutes. Watch them closely to prevent burning.

Nutrition's Fact: Calories 265, Carbohydrates 22g, Protein 29g, Fat 5g

Parmesan-Roasted Cauliflower

Preparation Time: *20 Minutes Yield: 1 Serving*

Ingredients

- One head cauliflower, cut into small florets
- One teaspoon salt
- One teaspoon mixed herbs
- 1/2 teaspoon ground black pepper
- Three tablespoons olive oil
- 1/2 cup grated Parmesan cheese

Directions

- Preheat the oven carefully to 450 degrees F. Line a baking sheet with aluminum foil.
- Prepare the cauliflower on the prepared baking sheet. Sprinkle it with mixed herbs, salt, and pepper. Drizzle it with olive oil; toss it until well coated. Sprinkle Parmesan cheese on top.
- Roast in the preheated oven until crisp, 10 to 15 minutes.

Nutrition's Fact: Calories 264, Carbohydrates 20g, Protein 35g, Fat 4g

Creamy Keto Chicken-Poblano Soup

Preparation Time: *20 Minutes Yield: 1 Serving*

Ingredients

- Four skinless, boneless chicken thighs
- salt and ground black pepper to taste
- 10 ounces of water
- 10 ounces tomatoes with green chile peppers(diced)
- One poblano pepper, sliced
- 1/2 onion, diced
- 8 ounces cream cheese, softened

Directions

- Season the chicken thighs smoothly with salt and black pepper.
- Combine poblano pepper, water, tomatoes, and onion in a multi-functional pressure cooker. Combine chicken. Close and lock the lid. Prefer Meat setting and set the timer for 20 minutes. Allow 10 to 15 minutes for pressure to build.
- Release the pressure using the natural-release system according to the manufacturer's instructions for 5 minutes. Release the remaining force carefully using the quick-release method according to the manufacturer's directions, about 5 minutes. Open and separate the lid.
- Remove chicken from the pot and shred. Combine cream cheese to the soup in the pan and stir until mixed well. Return shredded chicken to the bowl and mix well.

Nutrition's Fact: Calories 261, Carbohydrates 19g, Protein 31g, Fat 3g

One-Pan Keto Shrimp and Asparagus

Preparation Time: *20 Minutes Yield: 1 Serving*

Ingredients

- One tablespoon avocado oil
- Two tablespoons butter
- Two teaspoons minced garlic
- 3/4 pound jumbo shrimp
- salt to taste
- 1/2 teaspoon red pepper flakes
- 1/2 bunch fresh asparagus, trimmed
- ground black pepper to taste
- One medium lemon halved
- 1/4 cup finely shredded Parmesan cheese

Directions

- Heat the avocado oil and butter together in a skillet over medium temperature. Combine garlic and cook until lightly browned for 5 minutes. Place the shrimp into one side of the pan; season it with salt and red pepper flakes. Combine asparagus to the other bottom of the pan and season it with salt and black pepper. Flip the shrimp after about 2 minutes and roll asparagus over, squeeze lemon juice on top of shrimp, and proceed cooking about 5 minutes more. Smoothly sprinkle Parmesan cheese over shrimp. Shift to a plate and pour pan juices over shrimp.

Nutrition's Fact: Calories 215, Carbohydrates 25g, Protein 36g, Fat 2g

Keto Lemon-Garlic Chicken Thighs

Preparation Time: *20 Minutes Yield: 1 Serving*

Ingredients

- 1/4 cup lemon juice
- Two tablespoons olive oil
- One teaspoon Dijon mustard
- Two cloves garlic, minced
- 1/4 teaspoon salt
- 1/8 teaspoon ground black pepper
- Four skin-on, bone-in chicken thighs
- Four lemon wedges

Directions

- Whisk lemon juice, olive oil, Dijon mustard, garlic, salt, and pepper together in a bowl. Set the marinade aside.
- Place the chicken thighs carefully into a resealable plastic bag. Pour the marinade over the chicken and seal the bag, making positive to cover all parts of the chicken. Refrigerate for at least 2 hours.
- Preheat an air fryer carefully to 360 degrees F.
- Separate chicken from marinade and pat dry with paper towels. Place chicken parts in the air fryer basket, cooking in batches if needed.
- Fry it until chicken is no longer pink at the bone and the juices run clear 25 minutes. An instant-read thermometer entered near the bone should read 165 degrees F. Squeeze a lemon wedge over each piece upon serving.

Nutrition's Fact: Calories 260, Carbohydrates 18g, Protein 30g, Fat 2g

Keto Spaghetti Squash Carbonara

Preparation Time: *20 Minutes Yield: 1 Serving*

Ingredients

- One spaghetti squash, halved and seeded
- Three slices of bacon
- One teaspoon minced garlic
- Two eggs
- 1/4 cup grated Parmesan cheese
- 1/4 cup chopped parsley
- salt and ground black pepper to taste

Directions

- Preheat the oven carefully to 400 degrees F (200 degrees C) — line a baking sheet with parchment paper; place the squash on top, cut-side down.
- Bake in the preheated oven until skin is easily pierced with a fork, about 45 minutes.
- While squash is cooking, fry bacon in a large skillet over medium-high heat until crisp, 15 minutes. Shift it to a paper towel-lined plate, reserving grease in the skillet. Crumble bacon when cool enough to handle.
- Freshly baked squash until easily handled. Scrape flesh into noodles using a fork. Place the noodles and garlic in the skillet with the reserved bacon grease. Cook it over medium heat for 5 minutes; reduce heat to low.
- Whisk the eggs and Parmesan cheese together in a small bowl; add to skillet and mix continuously for 5 minutes. Remove it from temperature and stir in cooked bacon pieces, parsley, salt, and pepper. Serve immediately.

Keto Bacon Cheeseburger Soup

Preparation Time: *20 Minutes Yield: 1 Serving*

Ingredients

- Six slices bacon
- 1 pound lean ground beef (80% lean)
- 3 cups reduced-sodium beef broth
- 1 cup shredded Cheddar cheese
- 4 ounces cream cheese
- Two spears kosher dill pickles, chopped
- Three tablespoons tomato paste
- One tablespoon steak sauce
- Two teaspoons spicy brown mustard
- One teaspoon onion powder
- One teaspoon chili powder
- One teaspoon ground black pepper
- One head of romaine lettuce, chopped into bite-sized pieces
- Six grape tomatoes halved
- 1/4 cup chopped red onion

Directions

- Heat a large soup pot over medium-high temperature and add bacon. Cook until crisp, about 15 minutes. Transfer to a paper towel-lined plate. Set aside to cool.
- Combine the beef to the soup pot and flatten with a spatula. Cook until the bottom is browned, about 5 minutes. Flip and cook another side, about 5 minutes more. Combine broth, Cheddar cheese, cream cheese, pickles, tomato paste, steak sauce, mustard, onion powder, chili powder, and black pepper. Mix it well to combine, breaking meat into smaller pieces.

- Reduce heat to low; cook it and stir until cream cheese has melted for about 5 minutes. Cover it and cook the soup for 25 minutes more.
- Ladle soup into individual bowls. Divide lettuce between bowls and fold into the soup. Crumble one slice of cooked bacon into each bowl and garnish with tomatoes and red onion.

Nutrition's Fact: Calories 263, Carbohydrates 19g, Protein 33g, Fat 1g

Cheesy Cauliflower Risotto with Bacon

Preparation Time: *20 Minutes Yield: 1 Serving*

Ingredients

- Four bacon strips, diced
- 1 cup diced baby Bella mushrooms
- 1/2 white onion, diced
- Three cloves garlic, minced
- 1 (16 ounces) package frozen riced cauliflower
- 1 cup chicken stock
- 1 1/2 cups grated Parmesan cheese
- 1 cup heavy cream

Directions

- Heat a large saucepan over medium-high temperature. Combine bacon and cook until crisp, 10 minutes. Remove the bacon using a slotted spoon and transfer to a small bowl.
- Add onion, mushrooms, and garlic to the bacon fat. Saute until softened and gently browned, about 5 minutes. Combine cauliflower rice and chicken stock and mix it well. Let them simmer until cauliflower rice has absorbed most of the capital, about 10 minutes.
- Stir it in Parmesan cheese and heavy cream; mix it properly. Pulse a few times utilizing an immersion blender to cut down any large pieces. Cook until heated it through, about 10 minutes. Stir it in about 3/4 of the cooked bacon. Shift the risotto to a serving bowl and top with the remaining bacon.

Nutrition's Fact: Calories 262, Carbohydrates 21g, Protein 34g, Fat 4g

Asparagus-Spinach-Artichoke Casserole

Preparation Time: *20 Minutes Yield: 1 Serving*

Ingredients

- 2 (15 ounce) cans asparagus, drained
- 1 (6.5 ounces) jar marinated artichoke hearts, drained
- 13.5 ounces spinach
- 1 (4 ounces) can sliced mushrooms
- 1 cup heavy whipping cream
- 1 (8 ounces) package cream cheese
- 1/2 cup vegetable broth
- 1/2 teaspoon dried Italian seasoning
- 1/2 teaspoon garlic powder
- 1 (8 ounces) package cream cheese
- 1/2 (8 ounces) package sharp Cheddar cheese

Directions

- Spread the asparagus across the bottom of a 9x13-inch casserole dish. Scatter artichoke hearts on top. Put the casserole dish in the oven; this will remove some residual moisture from the vegetables as the oven heats.
- Preheat the oven carefully to 350 degrees F (175 degrees C).
- Place the spinach and mushrooms in a microwave-safe bowl. Heat in microwave until moisture evaporates, about 10 minutes.
- Transfer the spinach and mushrooms into a pot over medium heat. Add heavy cream, cream cheese, and broth. Cook it and stir until cream cheese melts and sauce thickens about 5 minutes. Reduce heat to low. Stir it in Italian seasoning and garlic powder; cook until flavors meld, about 3 minutes.

- Remove casserole from the oven; pour the sauce over the vegetables. Top it with Cheddar cheese slices.
- Bake it in the preheated oven until the top has lightly browned and the edges are crumbly about 20 minutes. Let it cool properly for about 10 minutes before serving.

Nutrition's Fact: Calories 264, Carbohydrates 22g, Protein 31g, Fat 6g

Low-Carb Keto Cheese Taco Shells

Preparation Time: *20 Minutes Yield: 1 Serving*

Ingredients

- 2 cups shredded Cheddar cheese

Directions

- Preheat the oven carefully to 400 degrees F (200 degrees C) — line 2, baking the sheets with parchment paper or silicone mats.
- Then wrap the handle of a wooden spoon with aluminum foil — the balance between 2 tall cans is balanced.
- Spread the Cheddar cheese on the prepared baking sheets into four 6-inch rounds placed 2 inches apart.
- Bake it in the preheated oven until cheese melts and is gently brown, 6 to 8 minutes. Cold for 5 minutes. Lift it with a spatula and drape over the wrapped wooden handle; cold until set, about 10 minutes.

Nutrition's Fact: Calories 268, Carbohydrates 24g, Protein 33g, Fat 3g

Coconut Fat Bombs

Preparation Time: *20 Minutes Yield: 1 Serving*

Ingredients

- 1/2 cup coconut oil
- 2 cups unsweetened coconut
- Two tablespoons honey
- 1/3 teaspoon vanilla extract
- One tablespoon dark chocolate chips

Directions

- Place coconut oil in a microwave-safe bowl; warm in the microwave, about 5 minutes. Stir it in honey, coconut, and vanilla extract. Form it into balls and place it on a freezer-safe plate. Freeze until solid, about 10 minutes.
- While fat bombs are chilling, soften chocolate chips in a microwave-safe bowl in the microwave, about 1 minute. Drizzle the melted chocolate over fat bombs. Return to the freezer until chocolate has set, about 15 minutes more.

Nutrition's Fact: Calories 265, Carbohydrates 22g, Protein 29g, Fat 5g

Sheet Pan Lemon Garlic Salmon with Asparagus

Preparation Time: *20 Minutes Yield: 1 Serving*

Ingredients

- cooking spray
- 2 (1 pound) salmon fillets
- 1 pound fresh thin asparagus, trimmed
- Three tablespoons olive oil
- Three tablespoons lemon juice
- Four cloves garlic, minced
- Two teaspoons sea salt
- One teaspoon ground black pepper
- One lemon, sliced into rounds

Directions

- Preheat the oven carefully to 350 degrees F. Line a rimmed 9x12-inch baking sheet with parchment paper and grease it with cooking spray place the salmon fillets and asparagus in a single layer.
- Stir the olive oil, lemon juice, and garlic in a bowl. Drizzle the garlic mix over salmon and asparagus — season with salt and pepper place lemon rounds on top.
- Bake it in the preheated oven until salmon flakes directly with a fork, 15 to 20 minutes.

Nutrition's Fact: Calories 264, Carbohydrates 20g, Protein 35g, Fat 4g

Best Keto Bread Rolls

Preparation Time: *20 Minutes Yield: 1 Serving*

Ingredients

- cooking spray
- 1 1/2 cups blanched almond flour
- Five tablespoons psyllium husk
- One teaspoon sea salt
- 1 cup boiling water
- Three egg whites
- Two teaspoons white vinegar
- Two tablespoons sesame seeds

Directions

- Preheat the oven carefully to 350 degrees F (175 degrees C) — grease a baking sheet with cooking spray.
- Combine almond flour, psyllium husk, and salt in a bowl; mix well. Add water, egg whites, and vinegar; whisk with an electric mixer until well combined, and a thick dough has formed about 1 minute.
- Wet your hands and shape dough into eight rolls. Arrange rolls on the prepared baking sheet. Sprinkle sesame seeds on top.
- Bake it properly in the preheated oven until golden, about 55 minutes.

Nutrition's Fact: Calories 261, Carbohydrates 19g, Protein 31g, Fat 3g

Keto Tortillas

Preparation Time: *20 Minutes Yield: 1 Serving*

Ingredients

- 1 cup blanched almond flour
- Three tablespoons coconut flour
- Two teaspoons xanthan gum
- One teaspoon baking powder
- One pinch salt
- Two teaspoons apple cider vinegar
- One egg
- Three tablespoons water
- cooking spray

Directions

- Combine xanthan gum, baking powder, almond flour, coconut flour, salt in the bowl of a food processor; pulse until well combined. Pour apple cider vinegar into the mix and blend until smooth. Add egg and water, one tablespoon at a time, and mix until a sticky dough ball has formed. Put the dough on a surface moistened with almond flour, and knead until smooth, about 5 minutes. Cover the dough in plastic wrap and then let it stand for 15 minutes. Divide dough into eight equal balls; roll out each ball into a 5-inch disc between two parchment paper sheets.
- Heat an iron skillet over medium-high temperature and grease with cooking spray. Place the dough disc in the hot skillet for just 5 seconds; flip it quickly with a spatula, and cook until effortlessly golden, about 45 seconds. Flip and cook it for another 40 seconds.

Simple Keto Zucchini Hash

Preparation Time: *20 Minutes Yield: 1 Serving*

Ingredients

- Four small zucchini, grated and squeezed dry
- Three tablespoons coconut oil
- One tablespoon butter
- 1/3 cup grated Parmesan cheese
- One teaspoon chili powder, or more to taste
- One teaspoon sea salt
- One teaspoon cayenne pepper (optional)
- Two eggs, beaten

Directions

- Combine the zucchini with coconut oil and butter in a skillet over medium heat. Combine chili powder, salt, Parmesan cheese, and cayenne pepper. Mix until cheese melts.
- Reduce temperature to low and add eggs; stir quickly until thoroughly mixed. Increase temperature back to medium and cook, mixing and occasionally flipping until the hash's edges have lightly browned about 15 minutes.

Nutrition's Fact: Calories 260, Carbohydrates 18g, Protein 30g, Fat 2g

Keto Diet Avocado Egg Bake

Preparation Time: *20 Minutes Yield: 1 Serving*

Ingredients

- One avocado halved and pitted
- Two eggs
- 1/4 cup shredded Cheddar cheese
- salt and freshly ground black pepper
- One tablespoon chopped fresh parsley, or to taste (optional)

Directions

- Preheat the oven carefully to 425 degrees F (220 degrees C).
- Scoop out a little of the avocado from where the pit was to make room for one egg. Place on a baking sheet and crack one egg on top of each avocado half.
- Bake in the preheated oven until the egg has cooked, 15 to 20 minutes. Spray Cheddar cheese on top and season with salt and pepper. Garnish it with fresh parsley.

Nutrition's Fact: Calories 261, Carbohydrates 17g, Protein 31g, Fat 5g

Keto Bacon-Wrapped Asparagus with Lemon Aioli

Preparation Time: *20 Minutes Yield: 1 Serving*

Ingredients

- 3/4 cup mayonnaise
- One teaspoon Dijon mustard
- One clove garlic, minced
- One teaspoon lemon zest
- One tablespoon fresh lemon juice
- 1/4 teaspoon garlic salt
- One bunch of fresh asparagus, trimmed
- Ten slices bacon
- olive oil cooking spray
- One pinch cracked black pepper

Directions

- Combine mayonnaise, Dijon mustard, garlic, lemon zest, lemon juice, and garlic salt in a bowl and mix well. Refrigerate lemon aioli until ready to use.
- Preheat an outdoor grill for medium temperature and lightly oil the grate.
- Divide asparagus stalks into groups of 6 stems, depending on the thickness of the asparagus. Wrap each asparagus bundle tightly with one piece of bacon, overlapping as you wrap and tucking the ends under the bacon so it holds securely.
- Place the asparagus bundles in a single layer on a piece of aluminum foil. Spray packets lightly with olive oil spray and top the bacon with cracked pepper.

- Grill the asparagus bundles on the foil for 10 minutes. Flip each packet and grill until the bacon has cooked through and crisp, an additional 10 minutes. Serve with lemon aioli.

Nutrition's Fact: Calories 263, Carbohydrates 19g, Protein 33g, Fat 1g

Keto Cocoa Mug Cake

Preparation Time: *20 Minutes Yield: 1 Serving*

Ingredients

- Six tablespoons almond flour
- Two tablespoons unsweetened cocoa powder
- Two teaspoons low-calorie natural sweetener
- 1/2 teaspoon baking powder
- 1/8 teaspoon salt
- Two eggs
- Two tablespoons coconut oil, melted

Directions

- Mix the almond flour, cocoa powder, sweetener, baking powder, and salt in a small bowl.
- Beat eggs in a bowl using an electric mixer until light and fluffy. Slowly combine melted coconut oil and beaten eggs to the almond flour mixture, fluttering everything together with a fork.
- Carefully grease two microwave-safe mugs. Pour batter into cups, leaving at least 1 inch of space at the top so the cakes can rise.
- Microwave on high power for 5 minutes. Test cakes for doneness. Maintain cooking in 10 second-intervals, if necessary, until patties are cooked through and not runny in the middle.

Nutrition's Fact: Calories 262, Carbohydrates 21g, Protein 34g, Fat 4g

Keto Pepperoni Pizza with Fathead Crust

Preparation Time: *20 Minutes Yield: 1 Serving*

Ingredients

- Two teaspoons yeast
- Two tablespoons warm water
- 3 cups shredded part-skim mozzarella cheese
- One large egg, lightly beaten
- 1 cup almond flour
- One teaspoon xanthan gum
- 1 or 4 cups no sugar added pizza sauce
- 1/8 teaspoon salt
- 2 ounces sliced pepperoni
- One pinch of red pepper flakes to taste (optional)

Directions

- Preheat the oven carefully to 375 degrees F (190 degrees C). Line a baking sheet with parchment paper.
- Mix the yeast into warm water in a small cup, stirring to dissolve. Set aside.
- Place 1 or 2 cups mozzarella cheese into a medium microwave-safe bowl — microwave for 90 seconds, stirring every 25 seconds until thoroughly melted. Stir it in the yeast mixture and egg; stir to mix. The dough will not mix well at this point.
- Stir in xanthan gum, almond flour, and salt. If difficult to blend, reheat in the microwave for 25 seconds to soften the cheese. Stir again until well incorporated. Knead dough by hand for 5 minutes.
- Place the mixture on the cooled baking sheet and press with your fingers into a thin crust 12 to 13 inches in diameter.

- Bake in the preheated oven until gently browned, about 10 minutes — spread pizza sauce over pizza. Top with remaining 1 or 2 cups mozzarella cheese, next scatter pepperoni on top.
- Return to the oven and bake it until cheese has melted, about 5 minutes more. Sprinkle with red pepper flakes. Cut into six slices.

Nutrition's Fact: Calories 264, Carbohydrates 22g, Protein 31g, Fat 6g

7 Days Meal Plan

Day-1

Breakfast: Garlic Tuscan Chicken

Lunch: Keto Chicken Parmesan

Dinner: Sausage, Zucchini, and Cauli Keto Risotto

Day-2

Breakfast: Keto Beef Egg Roll Slaw

Lunch: Keto Smoky Chicken With Vegetable

Dinner: Creamy Keto Cauliflower Risotto

Day-3

Breakfast: Creamy Keto Taco Soup with Ground Beef

Lunch: Keto Smothered Chicken Thighs

Dinner: Ultimate Low-Carb Zucchini Lasagna

Day-4

Breakfast: Keto Chicken and Kale Stew

Lunch: Keto Brownies

Dinner: Basic Keto Cheese Crisps

Day-5

Breakfast: Easy Keto Alfredo Sauce

Lunch: Simple Cauliflower Keto Casserole

Dinner: Low-Carb Almond Cinnamon Butter Cookies

Day-6

Breakfast: Keto Low-Carb Lemon Poppy Seed Muffins

Lunch: Keto Cheesecake Cupcakes

Dinner: Fluffy Keto Pancakes

Day-7

Breakfast: Roasted Brussels Sprouts

Lunch: Low-Carb Bacon Cheeseburger Casserole

Dinner: Keto Shrimp Scampi with Broccoli Noodles

Conclusion

Essentially, it is a diet that allows the body to release ketones into the bloodstream. Most cells tend to use blood sugar from carbohydrates as the body's key source of nutrition. In the absence of circulating blood sugar from food, we continue to break down accumulated fat into molecules called ketone bodies (the process is called ketosis). When you achieve ketosis, most cells can use ketone to produce energy before consuming carbohydrates again. The transition from circulating glucose to the breakdown of accumulated fat as a source of energy typically occurs over two to four days of eating less than 20 to 50 grams of carbohydrate per day. Bear in mind that this is a highly individualized procedure, and some people require a more limited diet to start producing enough ketones. A ketogenic diet can be an exciting approach to treating such diseases and may improve weight loss. Yet, it's hard to follow because it can be high on red meat and other unhealthy, refined, and salty foods that are famously unhealthful. We don't know anything about the long-term consequences, presumably because it's so hard to stick with that people can't eat that way for a long time.

Thank you for choosing and reading this book

Michelle J. Griffin

"Did this book help you in some way? If so, I'd love to hear about it. Honest reviews help readers find the right book for their needs."

Check out my books!

Search on amazon Michelle J. Griffin

Out now:

The Complete Guide To Wellness in All Dimensions

How to Understand and Control Your Wellness to Live a Happy Life and Healthy Life

LEARN HOW TO ACHIEVE ALL FORMS OF WELNESS

This book focuses on practicing healthy habits that will help you improve your physical and mental state. By taking time to learn about wellness in all aspects (maybe while sipping a cup of tea), you will be able to live a healthy and fulfilling life. This book touches all aspects of wellness; that is the physical, emotional, social, environmental, intellectual, occupational, financial and spiritual aspect of wellness individually so that readers will have the incredible experience of connecting to their selves in the deepest way to create balance in their life.

Drawing on information from research and her own personal experiences and opinions, Michelle J Griffin creates an educative book for people who worry about their wellbeing. this beautiful book will help readers reflect on their past choice and work on their personal growth by figuring out the wellness aspects they have flourished in and the ones that they have ignored.

What readers will reach from this book includes but is not limited to a sample wellness plan, clear instructions to help you successfully achieve all forms of wellness, information on the benefits of all aspects of wellness, comparisons of how some forms of wellness are intertwined, motivation quotes from different genres and a scientific, fun and logical written manual on how to guide your wellness growth.

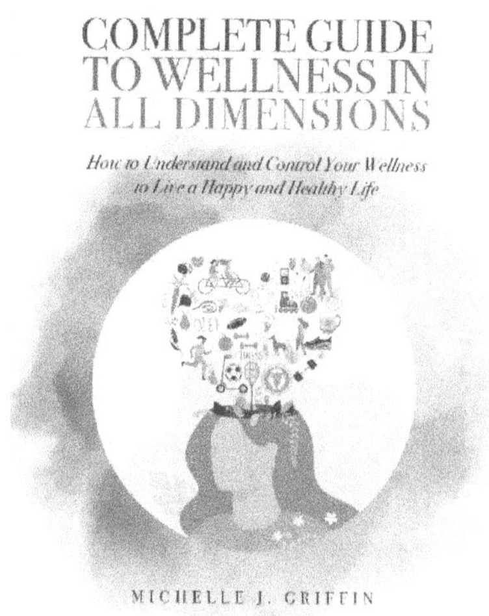

Thank you

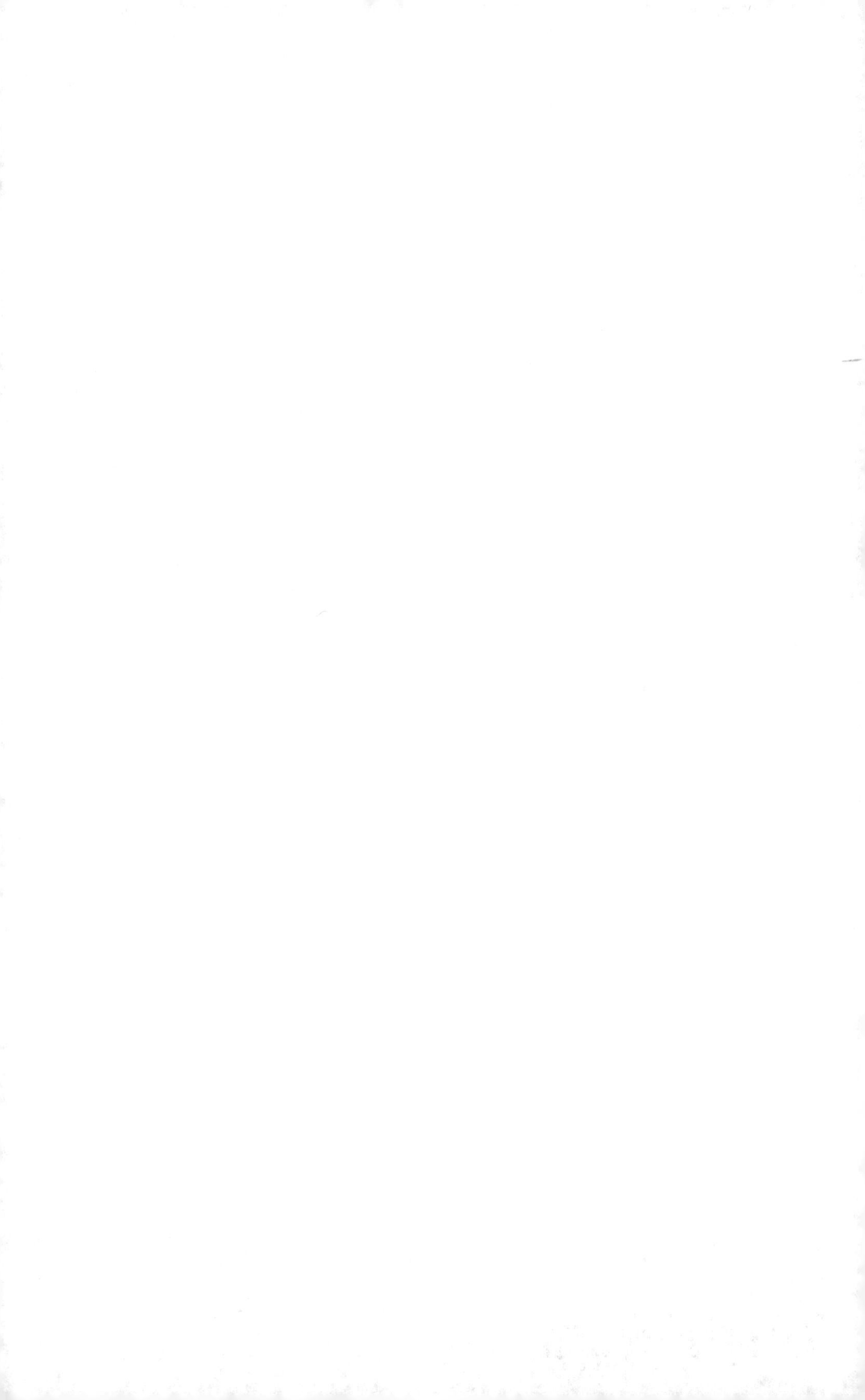